Private Medical Practice

Christopher Locke

Industrial Relations Officer, British Medical Association, and
formerly Secretary of the Private Practice and Professional Fees
Committee, British Medical Association

with a Foreword by
David E Pickersgill

Chairman of the Private Practice and Professional Fees Committee,
British Medical Association

Radcliffe Medical Press
Oxford and New York

© 1994. Radcliffe Medical Press Ltd
15 Kings Meadow, Ferry Hinksey Road, Oxford OX2 0DP, UK

141 Fifth Avenue, Suite N, New York, NY 10010, USA

British Library Cataloguing in Publication Data

A cataloguing record for this book is available from the British Library.

ISBN 1 870905 99 7

Contents

Foreword

During his time as Secretary to the Private Practice and Professional Fees Committee of the BMA, Christopher Locke acquired a vast amount of knowledge about the problems and difficulties experienced by doctors who were engaged in private practice. Many of these difficulties arise because private practice and its special problems are not subjects covered in any medical curriculum and little information about private practice is passed on to doctors in training grades. It is only when newly appointed consultants or principals in general practice actually start to practise that they become aware of the gaps in their knowledge in this important area of medical practice.

This book provides a comprehensive guide to all aspects of private practice and contains a wealth of information about equipment and the complexities of taxation and pension arrangements. There is a useful review of the arrangements in the UK for private medical practice and the book concludes with some thoughts about how private practice may develop in the future and the impact of various social and political factors on this development.

The text should form an invaluable source of reference, not only for new entrants to consultant and general practice, but also for those who have been established for some years and who may wish to update their knowledge on particular areas of private practice.

David E Pickersgill
January 1994

Acknowledgements

I am grateful for the support and encouragement given to this venture by colleagues in the British Medical Association, both elected representatives and staff. I should especially like to thank Dr David Pickersgill, Chairman of the Private Practice and Professional Fees Committee, and his deputy chairman, Mr Richard Marcus FRCS, for their help in making this book possible. I am grateful also for the inspiration and encouragement of Mr Norman Ellis, head of the BMA's Contractor Services Division.

I would like to take the opportunity of thanking all of the following who have assisted with comments and assistance with the diverse areas covered by the book: Sally Watson, Secretary, Central Consultants and Specialists Committee; Jon Ford, BMA Economist; Ann Sommerville, Executive Secretary, Medical Ethics Committee; Roger Dowsett, Solicitor; John Dean, Pannell Kerr Foster; and Douglas Shields, Medical Insurance Agency.

My grateful thanks also go to Helena Morris, Janet Whitehouse and Lisa Parker for their diligence and patience in typing the manuscript.

The book is affectionately dedicated to my wife Kaye and our daughters Helen and Corinne.

Introduction

The term 'private medical practice' can be defined very broadly. However, in this book it refers principally to the treatment of private patients. Therefore the book does not attempt to examine in great detail the full range of private medical services currently provided in this country; nor is it a clinical textbook.

The objectives of the book are threefold: first, to explain the rules which govern the practice of treating private patients; secondly, to offer practical advice to those thinking of setting up in private medical practice for the first time; and finally, to describe the various permutations of private medical practice and to speculate about its future development.

The book will therefore be of most relevance to hospital specialists, but it should also be of interest to general practitioners and to all those wishing to understand private practice and the workings of the private healthcare 'industry' in the UK.

At the time of writing, little statistical research was available on the activities and earnings of private practitioners. The survey of private specialists' fees undertaken by the Monopolies and Mergers Commission in 1993 is expected to provide the first extensive 'hard' data on these matters. The final report of the enquiry was not available, however, when this book went to press. The author has, therefore, to some extent anticipated that report's conclusions.

As well as providing explanations and advice, the book contains opinions on matters on which, in the absence of factual data, there may not be a consensus. The opinions expressed on such matters are those of the author, and should not be assumed to be those of either the British Medical Association or any other individuals with whom he may be associated.

Christopher Locke
April 1994

1

Medical Practice in the UK: An Overview

Interdependence of public and private healthcare provision

In order to understand the nature of private medical practice in the UK it is essential to appreciate the symbiotic relationship between public and private healthcare provision. There are two aspects to this relationship. The first is the extent to which the perceived failings of the National Health Service (NHS) define the parameters of the market in private healthcare. The second is the fact that, because the vast majority of the doctors who undertake private treatment also work in the NHS, the medical culture of the private sector and its modus operandi are, to a large extent, determined by that prevailing in the State system. These statements will require some explanation. In order to give this it will first be necessary to consider, in brief, the essential features of the NHS and how these affect its interrelationship with the private sector.

The National Health Service

Established by a Labour government in 1948, the NHS is a comprehensive healthcare system funded exclusively by taxation. It aims to provide free access to health services at the point of delivery to all UK citizens. It has proved to be a remarkably durable and popular institution. Despite its perceived failings, it has survived the stresses and strains of economic and political change during the last 45 years and continues to provide for the medical needs of the vast majority of British citizens 'from the cradle to the grave'. This is not the occasion to open up the debate about how it is funded. However it is of note that the system, often considered by its critics to be cumbersome, bureaucratic and wasteful of resources (it is the largest employer in Western Europe), continues to consume less than 6% of the UK's gross national product.

As we will see, the success of the NHS has had the effect of limiting the size of the market in private healthcare. Currently only about 12% of the UK population are covered by some form of private health insurance. The existence of a universal 'safety net', providing ready access to primary care and immediate emergency access to secondary care services, obviates the necessity for all-embracing health insurance and has limited the demand for private services to the areas where NHS provision is overused and in greatest demand. These are the acute specialties, particularly elective surgery. ('Acute' conditions are those which cause discomfort and require treatment but are not usually life-threatening. Among the most common are hernia repairs, varicose veins, extraction of wisdom teeth and hip replacements.)

The significance of NHS waiting-lists

The reasons why individuals opt for private treatment are many and various. 'Cultural' factors often play a part, as does the desire for comfort and privacy and the personal attention of a private doctor. In the opinion of many commentators, however, one of the most significant factors in recent years has been concern about the length of time the individual may have to wait for operative treatment on the NHS. While estimates vary, at least 70% of private treatment is accounted for by private medical insurance. According to Laing (1993), 'waiting for elective surgery under the NHS is at the heart of decisions to purchase private medical insurance'.

All elective procedures can be performed within the NHS but, despite an increase in the proportion of booked cases (ie those who are given a firm date of admission), it is generally not possible for patients to choose the date of admission, and they will have little choice in the location or timing of that treatment. Going private ensures early admission at a time and place convenient to the patient.

In fact the public perception of extensive waiting-times for surgery on the NHS in recent years is not supported by the evidence. According to the most recent available statistics, the median waiting-time for NHS elective surgery is only about six weeks. This is rather shorter than was the case 20 years ago. However, the figures suggest that there is a substantial pool of 'slow stream' patients who are having to wait considerably longer than the median: about 25% of patients awaiting elective surgery may have to wait in excess of one year, despite government-sponsored initiatives to reduce NHS waiting-lists. Whatever the truth of the public's perception of the waiting-list crisis it has led to a situation where the private services of consultants in acute specialties (where lengthy waiting-lists exist) have become a valued commodity.

The fact that the private sector now accounts for 20–25% of elective surgery carried out in the UK demonstrates that the private sector does, to some extent, relieve the pressure on the NHS by helping to reduce these waiting-lists in certain areas. This is an illustration of the mutual interdependence referred to above.

Of course the 'waiting-list factor' does not apply universally and there are notable exceptions. There are no waiting-lists in obstetrics, for instance, yet it rates as one of the most popular of the acute specialties in which private treatment is sought.

The concentration of private healthcare provision

In addition to the elective treatments described above, the private sector provides a number of specialist services which are either not available within the NHS or are provided only on a limited scale. These include cosmetic surgery, abortions, fertility treatment and various screening and diagnostic services. However, these are not normally covered by health insurance; nor are specialties catering for long-term and chronic conditions, eg geriatrics and oncology. This is because the cost of such treatments would increase the premiums of health insurance to a level beyond the reach of the average subscriber. Health insurance does not provide either for the services of general practitioners (GPs). The reasons are explained in the next chapter, but essentially the demand has been limited by the existence of universal free access to a network of NHS GPs and primary-care support services. Only those who are wealthy enough to pay for the additional benefits of a more personal service feel the need to have a private GP.

In terms of expenditure, private nursing and residential care is the largest element of private healthcare but the contribution of medical practitioners in this area is modest compared with the amount of private practice undertaken in acute hospitals.

Medical personnel

In the NHS, primary care is provided by a network of some 31 000 GPs, together with nurses, ancillary staff and co-workers; secondary care is provided by 19 000 hospital consultants, 31 000 doctors in less senior grades and a vast array of nurses, paramedics and support staff.

The numbers of patients seeking treatment from GPs privately is probably very small. Few NHS GPs have any private patients. However it has been estimated that about 12 000 NHS consultants undertake some degree of private practice and there may be as many as 6000 consultants who have retired from the NHS and practise privately on a part-time basis. There are no more than a few hundred wholly private doctors, both GPs and consultants, practising full-time; and almost all of these will have trained in the NHS.

In one sense the private sector can be regarded as parasitic on the NHS, in that it makes no effective contribution to the training of the medical personnel on whose services it relies, and makes only a small contribution to the training of nurses. However it may be said to subsidize the NHS in the manner in which the private practice fees paid to consultants allow them to maintain a high standard of income without any additional strain on the financial resources of their principal employer (*see* Chapters 5 and 7).

Very few doctors working in the private sector have salaried appointments (although there are some exceptions—eg doctors working in psychiatric hospitals and some other specialist units). Almost all work partially or mostly in the NHS.

Private medical care in the UK is provided via a contract (usually unwritten) between the patient and the private practitioner. It is rare (except with psychiatric treatment) for the institution where care is provided to be directly responsible for medical (as opposed to nursing) care. The choice of practitioner is determined by the system prevailing in the NHS.

Both from a strategic point of view, and from the point of view of the individual patient, the GP/consultant axis is the basis of healthcare delivery in the NHS. This has served as the model for the private sector. It may therefore be helpful to consider briefly the interrelationship of GP and consultant in the NHS and how this is translated into the private sector.

The role of the GP

The GP has accurately been described as the 'gatekeeper' of the NHS. What may not be obvious to outsiders is the extent to which he is a gatekeeper to private medicine also. General practice is acknowledged to be one of the strengths of the NHS and is justly described as a 'British success'. In almost no other developed nation has a system evolved which is so dependent on a network of primary-care practitioners. The effectiveness of this network helps to compensate for the fact that the UK has significantly fewer doctors per head of population than many of its EC partners.

The benefits of this system to the patient are obvious: the GP attends to all the minor medical complaints of his practice population, assesses their individual needs and co-ordinates provision of secondary care. The benefits to the system are equally clear: the GP ensures that only genuine calls are made on the more expensive secondary-care facilities. The GP's value lies in the ability to ration access to secondary care. The saving to the NHS is demonstrated by comparing costs with those of other healthcare systems in which direct access to secondary care is established.

Except for emergency treatment and certain non-life-threatening conditions, self-referral to secondary-care facilities is rare. In the wider interests of patient care, the General Medical Council actively discourages specialists from treating patients who have not been referred by a GP (*see* Chapter 2).

In all other forms of treatment the mechanism of referral is all-important. The GP determines which consultant to refer his patient to, and he is free to choose any consultant within or outside the local district. The GP's right to do so has been reinforced by successive government pronouncements, notwith-standing recent concern about the effect of 'extra-contractual referrals' in the post-reform NHS. When secondary treatment by the consultant of the GP's choice is completed, care of the patient is then transferred back to that GP. Thus the GP remains the guarantor of continuity of the patient's treatment.

Recently this pivotal role has been developed further, as part of the NHS re-forms, by making GPs responsible for their own budgets with which they may purchase secondary care for their patients. By giving GPs the right to 'shop around', the Conservative government has made them the instrument of their plans to bring market forces into play in the NHS. Fundholders are now also free to purchase healthcare directly from the private sector if this is a cheaper and more effective option for their patients.

The role of the consultant

The consultant has long been regarded as the pinnacle of hospital medicine. Though an employee of a health authority (or NHS Trust), he has a profes-sional contract which allows him to work flexibly and manage the treatment of the patients entrusted to his care as he sees fit. In return he assumes com-plete responsibility for the treatment of these patients.

Despite the introduction of clinical directorates, the consultant remains the prime mover and initiator of all hospital treatment. The clinical director is no more than 'primus inter pares'. However, the range of consultant activity is always constrained by budgetary considerations, which often bring the con-sultant into conflict with hospital administrators (both clinical directors and lay managers) who control the purse strings.

A key element of the contract, which testifies to its professional nature, is the consultant's ability to manage private and NHS patients simultaneously. The NHS consultant is usually permitted to manage as many private patients he feels able to treat, either in beds in the NHS hospital where he works or in his rooms or local private facilities, provided his private work does not inter-fere with the carrying out of his NHS duties (*see* Chapter 3).

Many fear that the introduction of locally devised Trust contracts for newly appointed consultants will lead to a gradual erosion of the flexibility with which consultants have traditionally been able to manage their time, though the freedom to undertake private practice under Trust contracts will inevitably vary.

The private patient 'compromise'

The simultaneous responsibility for both NHS and private patients owes its existence to a compromise patched together at the inception of the NHS. The Secretary of State for Health and architect of the NHS, Aneurin Bevan, encountered many difficulties in establishing a system which was acceptable to the medical profession. One of the points at issue during the long-drawn-out negotiations with the British Medical Association was the question of specialists' private patients. The chosen solution was, as Bevan put it, to 'stuff their mouths with gold'. This meant, among other things, allowing consultants to be able to continue treating their private patients, either in NHS beds or in private facilities, subject to availability.

From this compromise was born the maximum part-time contract and the very complex series of rules by which private practice is permitted to be undertaken in NHS hospitals (*see* Chapter 3). These were consolidated comparatively recently in the Department of Health document called the *Guide to the Management of Private Practice in Health Service Hospitals in England and Wales* (DHSS 1986, known colloquially as '*The Green Book*') and its equivalents in Scotland and Northern Ireland.

Restriction of opportunities for junior grades

Subject to occasional variations, the right to admit private patients to NHS hospitals has always been confined to doctors of consultant status. Junior hospital doctors are forbidden to undertake private practice other than outside their contracted hours, though they are obliged to assist consultants treating private patients in NHS hospitals for no additional remuneration. This has given rise to the feeling among junior grades that achievement of consultant status is a passport to greater financial rewards.

There has never been anything to prevent individuals who have not attained consultant status in the NHS from treating their own private patients (albeit outside NHS contracted time and with the approval of the consultant to whom they are responsible): but in practice the opportunities remain limited. The recognition accorded to NHS consultants by the health insurers has strengthened their pre-eminence. The creation within the NHS of a new grade of doctor, the associate specialist (AS), has done nothing to diminish this, as most health insurers will not accord specialist recognition to AS grade doctors. In practice the reliance on consultant status as the hallmark of the specialist means that the activities of even wholly private physicians and surgeons who have not held a substantive consultant post in the NHS are limited.

Access to private treatment

The benefits of the GP–consultant referral process were readily accepted by both patients and practitioners when it came to private treatment. The patient inevitably turned to his family doctor to suggest the name of a competent specialist when taking the decision to go private. The specialist, meanwhile, was content that the patient had been 'vetted' by a GP with whom he could correspond about the patient's treatment and to whom he could transfer aftercare responsibility.

This system was also readily embraced by the health insurers. The provident associations, some of whom predated the advent of the NHS and which continue to dominate the health insurance market (*see* Chapter 5), were mindful of the fact that, by ensuring that referral was 'necessary and appropriate', the GP would keep down their costs. They adapted their policies to the prevailing structure of the NHS by insisting on GP referral to named consultants or accredited specialists.

Where they parted company with the NHS was in being able to guarantee personal treatment by that specialist and not, as might be the case in the NHS, by his junior colleagues. This has been a mainstay and one of the major selling points of private treatment. The public were led to believe that private treatment guaranteed quality. While comfort and convenience were very important, the personal service of a top consultant was a significant consideration.

Specialist status and the health insurers

For many years the health insurers did not seek to influence in any way the choice of specialist treating their subscribers. They were content to let the patient's GP be the arbiter of the specialist's professional competence. However the last decade has seen the establishment of fairly strict criteria for recognition of specialist status by the health insurers. This usually involves reliance on the holding of a substantive NHS consultant post, or accreditation by the Royal Colleges or Joint Committees on Higher Specialist Training.

The establishment of these criteria was no doubt due to an emphasis on quality and the feeling that standards should be judged by qualifications, rather than just the subjective experience and opinions of GPs. As a result, a number of eminent practitioners have found themselves effectively 'derecognized'. The effect of non-recognition is to deny the patient reimbursement of the costs of any treatment carried out by that practitioner which, of course, can result in considerable difficulties for all concerned. The fact that 70% of private treatment is now accounted for by health insurance demonstrates how great an obstacle to successful private practice this can be.

The debate about specialist accreditation

Concern at the application of these criteria served to increase the groundswell of criticism of the system of specialist accreditation which was beginning to make itself felt in the early 1990s. The campaign to reform this system was given tremendous impetus by the government's acknowledgement in 1992 that the system was not in accord with the European Community directive on mutual recognition of specialist training. This acknowledgement led to the instigation of a fundamental review of specialist training by a working party headed by the government's chief medical officer, Dr Kenneth Calman. The review threatens to have enormously far-reaching implications both for the NHS and for private medical practice (see Chapters 3 and 18). However, for the present it is sufficient to note that the health insurers are still wedded to the system of accreditation established in and for the NHS, demonstrating once again how closely public and private healthcare provision in the UK are enmeshed.

The NHS reforms

The reform of the NHS initiated by the Conservative government, with the NHS and Community Care Act 1990, has involved the most radical shake-up in the provision of State healthcare since the foundation of the NHS. The creation of an internal market by means of a split between purchasers and providers, and the general break-up of the cumbersome regional and district administrative bureaucracy, have transformed the NHS beyond recognition. However, if critics of these reforms are to be believed, the overall effect may simply be to highlight even more starkly the gross underfunding which has lain at the root of the problems affecting the NHS since its inception.

Whether or not the reforms will be successful, the 1990s will certainly be tumultuous for the NHS and its medical personnel. The effects will, moreover, be carried over into the private sector, with private hospitals not knowing whether to expect an increase or decrease in demand for private services, and consultants not knowing whether they will enjoy greater or lesser freedom to undertake private practice in the post-reform regime. The distinction between the NHS and the private sector may become more blurred as a result of the reforms, but this will not necessarily work to the benefit of the medical profession. In any event, the concept of private practice as it is today may require complete redefinition in a few years' time.

With this proviso we will now consider the essential features of private medical practice as it exists today.

References and further reading

Calman K (1993) *Hospital Doctors: Training for the Future. Report of the Working Group on Specialist Medical Training.* DoH, London.

Central Consultants and Specialists Committee, BMA (1990) *The Consultant*

Handbook. BMA, London.

Department of Health and Social Security (1984) *Terms and Conditions of Service for Hospital Medical and Dental Staff*. DHSS, London.

Department of Health and Social Security (1986) *Guide to the Management of Private Practice in Health Service Hospitals in England and Wales*. DHSS, London.

General Medical Council (1992) *Professional Conduct and Discipline: Fitness to Practice*. GMC, London.

General Medical Services Committee, BMA (1983) *General Practice: A British Success*. BMA, London.

Grey-Turner E and Sutherland F W (1982) *A History of the British Medical Association, vol.II*. BMJ, London.

Laing W (1993) *Laing's Review of Private Healthcare*. Laing & Buisson, London.

National Audit Office (1989) *The NHS and Independent Hospitals*. HMSO, London.

Office of Health Economics (1992) *Compendium of Health Statistics 1992*. HMSO, London.

UK Health Departments/Joint Consultants Committee/Chairmen of Regional Health Authorities (1986) *Hospital Medical Staffing: Achieving a Balance*. DoH, London.

2

___

GPs and the Private Sector

NHS GPs

A considerable amount of private work is undertaken by full-time NHS GPs. The GP's NHS contract allows considerable flexibility, permitting private work—including treatment of private patients—to be undertaken in tandem with the doctor's NHS responsibilities. No figures are available regarding the amount of private fee-paid work undertaken by NHS GPs, nor of the number of private patients they may treat. A straw poll among any representative group of GPs is likely to indicate that only a minority have any private patients. In most cases, NHS GPs take on private patients only on request. They do not advertise for patients though they are now at liberty to do so, subject to the rules laid down by the General Medical Council (GMC) (*see* Chapter 8).

The significance of GP referral

A specialist is not obliged to refuse to treat a patient who has come to him directly seeking treatment without referral by his GP. However, few would ordinarily accept such patients in view of what the GMC says about this. Its guidance document *Professional Conduct and Discipline: Fitness to Practise* strongly supports GP referral as a means of protecting patients from potential exploitation, especially those rendered more susceptible through illness. The GP is seen to be the means by which the patient can obtain the most appropriate treatment from the most appropriate specialist.

There are several notable exceptions to this. GP referral is obviously not required in emergency situations. Treatment of foreign nationals who have no GP and come to this country seeking specialist private treatment may also be considered exempt, and the absence of GP referral is not regarded as an obstacle to treatment of certain types of non life-threatening conditions not covered by health insurance, including fertility treatment, abortion and cosmetic surgery.

The referral system is seen by the profession as the principal guarantee of continuity of care. Allowing one practitioner, the GP, to be fully appraised of the treatment received by his patient reduces the risk of the patient receiving treatment from several different specialists at once. Also, by having access to a patient's comprehensive medical record, the GP can communicate to the specialist at the time of referral any information which the specialist should know, including details of current treatment and medical history of which the patient may be unaware, have forgotten, remembered inaccurately or concealed. The conveying of accurate information on a 'need to know' basis protects the patient from inappropriate specialist advice and treatment.

Private referral by NHS GPs

Any doubts about the impartiality of GP advice on private specialist treatment will be allayed to some extent by the knowledge that the NHS GP derives no financial benefit from such referral. The reasons for this require detailed explanation.

The NHS GP is an independent contractor, not a salaried employee (his contract is a contract *for* services rather than a contract *of* service). The terms of this contract with the NHS (known perversely as the terms *of* service) require the GP to provide to the patients on his NHS list 'all necessary and appropriate general medical services' normally provided by general medical practitioners. These include referral to hospital services where he considers it necessary.

If secondary care is required, and the GP thinks that treatment can be obtained more quickly and at greater convenience to the patient if undertaken privately, he can refer his patient to a consultant privately (assuming his patient wants this and accepts that he must pay for the treatment). The GP does not *have* to refer privately, even when his patient requests it, if in his clinical opinion the patient's health would not be prejudiced by waiting for treatment on the NHS; but where he accepts that the patient would benefit from treatment provided via the private sector rather than the NHS, the GP has an obligation to refer the patient, with the patient's consent, to whichever private consultant the GP considers the most appropriate in the circumstances. It is not unusual for the patient to express a preference for a particular consultant which might differ from the GP's preferred choice, but in general it is better for both to agree on the choice.

The NHS GP is therefore obliged by his terms of service to refer his patients for treatment, either to the NHS or the private sector as appropriate. Logically, because this is a service which the NHS pays the GP to provide, he is forbidden to receive any additional money for this, either from the patient or anyone else (eg a health insurer, a private hospital or the consultant). This is, unfortunately, a sore point with many GPs. The consultant to whom referral is made will benefit financially from the referral but the GP will not.

Any attempt to obtain money from the GP's NHS patient in this respect would render the GP in breach of paragraph 38 of the terms of service— Schedule 2 to the NHS (General Medical Services) Regulations 1992—and lead to him having to account for his actions to a Service Committee of the Family Health Services Authority (FHSA). It is difficult to see, however, how the removal of this prohibition could be achieved without compromising the role of the GP as an independent and unbiased 'gatekeeper' and advocate of his patients' best interests. It could also be said to be in contravention of the GMC's guidance on financial interests (*see* Chapter 8).

GP validation of health insurance claims

When private treatment is carried out by a specialist, health insurers require claims by patients, for reimbursement or direct settlement of bills, to be authenticated or validated in some way. BUPA and PPP (*see* Chapter 5) normally regard the account of the specialist responsible, indicating the nature of treatment carried out, as sufficient validation—though on occasion they may require a more detailed report from the specialist. WPA and some other health insurers, on the other hand, specifically require claims to be validated by the referring GP.

There is an obvious logic to this. After all, the GP is independent of the specialist; he is the advocate of the patient; he is familiar with the case and will be in a position to judge whether the treatment required was necessary and carried out to his and the patient's satisfaction. The GP therefore operates in this context as a checking mechanism on the activities of the specialist. In rare cases BUPA and PPP may also have recourse to GP validation. Unfortunately, in no circumstances will any of the health insurers agree to pay the GP themselves for this service which, being entirely outside his NHS responsibilities, the GP is not obliged to undertake without payment.

Therefore in the vast majority of cases fees for validation fall, by default, upon the patient.* There is a logic in this also. Until the claim is authenticated, the health insurer has no obligation as regards the cost of the claim on its insurance, and it is up to the patient to prove that the claim is valid, incurring any expenditure involved therein entirely unsupported. GPs are at liberty to charge what they like for this service, though the BMA offers a suggested range of fees which is dependent on the scope of the work involved.

As we have noted, many GPs are resentful of the fact that they derive no financial benefit from effecting a private referral. Many would therefore regard a fee for validation as a means of recouping whatever expenditure they perceive to have been incurred. It is important to remember, however, that only a minority of claims under health insurance require GP validation and GPs cannot insist, as some have tried to do, on having forms returned to them by spe-

---

* At the time of writing the only exception to this involved policies provided by the Medical Insurance Agency (MIA) in conjunction with French insurance company Assurance Mutuelle Strasbourgeoise. In 1993 these companies announced that they would pay GPs £10.00 for each private treatment episode that they validated.

cialists for validation where it is not needed. Any GP who attempted such a course of action would quickly find himself in trouble. The provident associations are well aware of what GPs can and cannot do in this regard, and any unethical behaviour brought to their attention by a patient would be swiftly reported to the appropriate FHSA or the GMC.

Professional fees

There is a wide range of miscellaneous non-NHS services for which GPs are permitted to charge professional fees, under the broad headings listed in paragraph 38 of their terms of service. The major areas of this fee-paid work, such as medico-legal, insurance and occupational health work, are described in more detail in Chapter 17. These services may be provided either to individual patients or third parties. BMA members can obtain detailed advice on a whole range of these part-time medical services for which either suggested or negotiated rates of remuneration apply.

Paragraphs 51.16-51.17 and 52.19 of the Statement of Fees and Allowances (SFA) require that the amount of reimbursement allowed by the FHSA for premises rent/rates, and practice staff salaries, respectively, be abated when profits from private work exceed 10% of gross practice receipts. This is therefore a crucial consideration affecting the level of private practice undertaken by NHS GPs. It does not apply, however, to private work carried out other than at premises covered by rent and rates reimbursement or work which does not involve the practice staff whose salaries are being reimbursed. The definition of 'private income' given in paragraph 51.17 of the SFA is 'all professional income received from other than public sources'. It thus includes 'private fees received from NHS as well as private patients but excludes income from NHS hospitals, District Health Authorities and government departments'.

Where private work is undertaken solely in premises for which rent and rates reimbursement is received, a total of 10–20% of gross practice receipts being earned from private work will result in 10% abatement, where it represents 20–30%, the abatement will be 20%.

Where private work is undertaken partly in premises covered by rent and rates reimbursement and partly in premises not so covered, 15–20% of total gross practice receipts earned from private work will result in 10% abatement, and 25–30% in 20% abatement. As regards practice staff salary reimbursement, 10–20% of total gross practice receipts will result in 10% abatement, and 20–30% in 20% abatement. The same is true of locum allowances received during absence of a principal due to sickness.

Wholly private GPs

Any fully qualified medical practitioner can set up in private practice in the UK (*see* Chapter 7). The wholly private general practitioner does not need to have had any vocational training in general practice; he may have trained exclusively in hospital practice. However, many private GPs will have been vocationally trained in the NHS before confining themselves to private medicine. A number of such individuals will have continued with postgraduate education and may have become members and fellows of the Royal College of General Practitioners, for instance, after leaving the NHS. The only indication of the private GP's credentials is, as with any other doctor, the initials after his name.

The number of wholly private GPs remains small (only 324 in 1992 according to BMA figures). Wholly private GPs have traditionally been a disparate group, the previously restrictive rules of the GMC on advertising having prevented the establishment of any kind of central register. However, a new representative organization based in London, calling itself the Independent Doctors' Forum, has recently attempted to bring private GPs and specialists together and to establish such a register for circulation within the profession. (Their address can be found in the Appendix.)

Referral to the NHS by private GPs

Just as the NHS GP can refer to the private sector, the private GP can refer his patients to the NHS. The rationale for this is that, under the NHS, patients have a right to avail themselves of the services of an NHS GP. If they do not have one, however, and choose instead to pay for the services of a private GP, they still have an entitlement (as tax paying citizens) to NHS secondary-care services where these are required. Therefore, rather than to permit self-referral, the architects of the NHS accepted that private GPs would act as 'gatekeepers' to the NHS just like their NHS counterparts. It was consequently accepted as a principle that referral could be effected by any general practitioner. This applies to any out-patient service, including diagnostic tests (eg pathology and radiology).

The referral is treated exactly as if an NHS GP were involved, so the patient is treated in terms of clinical priority and the results of any tests should be returned to the private GP at no cost (Table 2.1). It is important to remember that it is the status and entitlement of the patient—not that of the doctor making the referral—which is all important in this situation. Many NHS managers are unaware of this principle which is clearly set out in paragraph 4.6 of *The Guide to the Management of Private Practice in NHS Hospitals in England and Wales*. (Similar provisions apply in Scotland and Northern Ireland.)

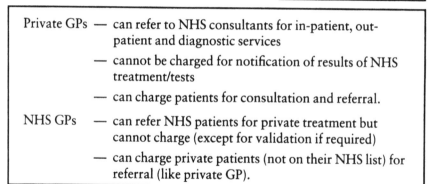

Private GPs	— can refer to NHS consultants for in-patient, out-patient and diagnostic services
	— cannot be charged for notification of results of NHS treatment/tests
	— can charge patients for consultation and referral.
NHS GPs	— can refer NHS patients for private treatment but cannot charge (except for validation if required)
	— can charge private patients (not on their NHS list) for referral (like private GP).

Table 2.1:   GP referral.

Why have both a private and an NHS GP?

A GP cannot treat the same patient privately and on the NHS at the same time. This is because the GP's terms of service forbid him to accept any remuneration in respect of patients for whose treatment he is responsible under the NHS. This prohibition extends to patients registered with partners within the same practice, presumably because of the conflict of interest which would arise if the GP were called upon to deputize for his partner and see that patient on the NHS. The practice has therefore grown up whereby some patients have both an NHS GP and a private one from a different practice. The reasons for remaining on the list of an NHS GP are twofold: because of the 'safety net' which the NHS provides as regards emergency treatment, and because of the cost of prescribing.

The private GP may well agree to be on call for his private patients, but he is not obliged to unless his contract with the patient specifically requires it. Other commitments may not always permit the GP to visit out of hours, especially if his private patient lives outside the area. It may then be advisable for a patient with a private GP to remain on an NHS GP's list, to call on that GP's services in an emergency.

Prescribing

The NHS GP can only provide an NHS prescription (FP10) to patients on his NHS list. He cannot prescribe on the NHS for his private patients, for whom he can provide private prescriptions only (the wholly private GP can only provide private prescriptions) (Table 2.2). Despite the fact that the standard prescription charge has increased considerably in recent years, many drugs are more costly 'over the counter' than when obtained on an NHS prescription. If the patient requires an expensive course of drugs, he is likely to prefer these to be prescribed by the NHS GP. Having two general practitioners is, however, not without its difficulties. Many NHS GPs will be unhappy at their patients having a private GP and may object to having to prescribe drugs when the patient has not consulted them previously about the treatment (*see* Chapter 8).

Private GPs	— cannot issue NHS prescriptions
	— can charge patients for prescriptions
NHS GPs	— cannot charge NHS patients for prescriptions (whether NHS or private)
	— cannot issue NHS prescriptions to private patients
	— can charge private patients (not on their NHS list) for prescriptions

Table 2.2: GP prescribing.

Managing private patients

Why, then, do patients choose to see a GP privately? In many cases it may be for the convenience of making greater demands on the doctor at times which suit them, and perhaps for the privilege of a second opinion and the opportunity to consult in confidence a practitioner other than the family's doctor.

The wholly private practitioner will clearly make a point of appearing attentive and responsive to his patient's needs. Many private GPs now provide a range of services equal to the best that the NHS can provide, including vaccinations, health screening, minor surgery and out-of-hours visits. Some have chosen to model the financing of their practice on the NHS, by asking patients to pay a weekly or annual registration fee with a small addition for visits and service such as certificates and vaccinations.

Most NHS GPs do not find it difficult to manage a small number of private patients on the same basis as those on their NHS list. Routine consultations and domiciliary visits will be arranged at a mutually convenient time outside normal surgery hours. Out-of-hours visits will be arranged to fit in with NHS calls, in order of clinical priority. It would of course be totally unethical to visit a private patient when a visit to an NHS patient in more urgent need was called for.

GPs and other health insurance matters

Private general practice remains the subject of a personal contract between the patient and doctor. As has been explained, the health insurers see little merit in offering to insure against the costs of private general practice because these costs are not great and because comparatively few people see the need to have a private GP. Recently, however, some insurance companies have shown interest in the idea. The French insurance company, Assurance Mutuelle Strasbourgeoise, has launched a policy which includes provision for private GP consultations, though it remains to be seen whether this will have popular appeal.

Of greater significance, perhaps, is the scheme run by Norwich Union Healthcare involving payment to GPs for minor surgery services. Because NHS GPs are forbidden to receive money for treating their own patients, this scheme involves payment for minor surgery, consistent with the list of minor surgical operations included in the NHS GP's terms of service, where it is undertaken by a practitioner other than the patient's own GP or partners. This has posed certain ethical questions (*see* Chapter 8). Other health insurers, including BUPA, have shown an interest in GP minor surgery, though only to the extent of considering the employment of GPs on sessional contracts to undertake such work in day case clinics attached to BUPA hospitals. If the insurers do eventually agree to forego total reliance on consultants for minor surgery, the opportunities for GPs in this area of the private sector are likely to increase.

Hotel work

One area of private practice, as opposed to private work, which is popular with GPs is the provision of GP services to hotel guests. Many large hotels will wish to have an arrangement with a local doctor to provide a 24-hour emergency service for their guests and staff. They may also be concerned to provide NHS services for resident staff, and require medical advice, similar to that provided to employers by occupational health doctors. Some hotel companies may therefore seek doctors who have an NHS list who are willing to provide an additional private service.

The arrangement will usually involve a retainer, paid monthly or annually by the hotel or its parent company to the doctor, plus item of service fees from private patients (the guests or staff requiring treatment). Often the doctor's bill will appear as part of the hotel bill. There are no ethical objections to this, provided there is no element of fee-splitting involved (*see* Chapter 8). However, it is essential that the doctor's bill is quite separate from the rest of the hotel bill and that no VAT or service charges are levied on it (medical services are exempt from VAT).

The GP will obviously have regard to the individual requirements of hotel guests. For example, American patients in particular will need details on the account for health insurance purposes. It is insufficient, for instance, simply to refer to 'medical professional services'. However, doctors should be wary when treating American patients, as medical malpractice suits are epidemic in the USA and the high level of compensatory awards may make it difficult for a UK defence organization to defend a doctor against whom such a claim is made.

To avoid misunderstandings, it is also essential for NHS GPs to become acquainted with the rules governing the provision of NHS services to overseas visitors, and to communicate an understanding of these rules to the management of the hotel with whom they have such a private arrangement.

GP treatment of overseas visitors

The treatment of overseas visitors is a subject which never ceases to confuse and concern doctors. The question of access to secondary care (ie hospital treatment) by overseas visitors is extremely complex; but, essentially, each case must be investigated and assessed by the relevant hospital authority whenever a call on those facilities is required. The provision of GP services is much simpler, though most NHS GPs will feel the need to obtain advice on the subject whenever a foreign national comes to them seeking treatment. They may be forgiven for being confused, as many of those who will have seen the Department of Health circular which governs these matters—HM(FP) (84)7—have assumed that the provision of NHS treatment will depend on such questions as whether the patient is ordinarily resident, or comes from the EC or a country with whom the UK has a reciprocal agreement.

In fact all references to such matters in the circular are largely irrelevant. Careful reading of the circular reveals that, except as regards emergency treatment, the NHS GP has complete discretion as to whether to treat a patient on the NHS as a temporary resident, or to refuse to treat him other than on a private basis. The circular makes it clear that many overseas visitors will expect to be asked to pay for medical treatment and the GP will not be committing any offence or breaching his terms of service in offering to treat them privately on any financial terms he and the patient can agree upon.

However, what the circular also makes clear is that *any* overseas patient, from any country, including those with whom the UK has no reciprocal agreement (eg the USA), can receive NHS treatment from a family doctor. The circular makes it clear that if no local GP is willing to treat the patient on the NHS, the patient can apply to the Family Health Services Authority which will allocate him to the list of a local GP. That GP will then be obliged to provide general medical services free of charge for the minimum number of days specified in the GP's terms of service. However, being assigned to an NHS GP's list does not give that patient any greater calling on NHS secondary-care services. Access to such services will depend on residency and country of origin.

Problems adduced by private GPs

A query frequently raised by private GPs concerns incapacity certificates. Many people assume that only NHS GPs can issue State incapacity certificates, MED 3 or MED 5, required for benefits payable by the Department of Social Security (DSS), but this is a fallacy. The DSS guidance booklet *Medical Evidence for Benefit Purposes* (DSS 1991) explicitly states that private practitioners are entitled to obtain supplies of these certificates for use in respect of their patients. The misapprehension may be due to the fact that NHS GPs traditionally obtain supplies of these certificates from their FHSA (which often has their stamp on them). In fact the FHSA is merely a distribution point and, according to the DSS guidance, private practitioners may themselves obtain supplies from the FHSA. In practice, however, few FHSAs are aware of this provision, and they may not easily be persuaded to make supplies available to private practitioners. The alternative is to obtain them from the DSS direct, although this is not always easy. If the local DSS office is unable to help, the DSS regional headquarters should still be able to provide the forms.

A further problem which has come to light recently concerns supplies of certain childhood vaccines (eg the polio vaccine), which, as a result of an arrangement between the suppliers and the Department of Health, can now only be obtained from health authorities. At the time of writing, the question of private practitioners' access to such supplies had not yet been sorted out.

Another area in which the Department of Health obviously overlooked the situation of wholly private GPs concerns the mechanism of referral to the NHS following the introduction of the purchaser/provider split as a consequence of the NHS and Community Care Act 1990. The advent of block contracts created the concept of 'extra-contractual referral' (ECR); with ECR came the standard referral letter, and the practice code number which enables hospitals to identify the source of a referral and determine whether it is part of a block contract or an ECR. The Department of Health decided that the practice code number should be based on the combination of the FHSA's own code number and the number allocated to each practice by the FHSA for reimbursement purposes. The wholly private practitioner will not have such a number, and when he refers patients to the NHS he might therefore have difficulty in persuading hospital staff that he does not have or need such a number. The DoH has now instructed hospitals to use the default code which they have for unidentified referrals in such eventualities. However, problems with this may still arise in certain areas.

What is also not entirely clear is whether such referrals to the NHS by private practitioners are always funded by the relevant district health authority. Do they fall to the budget of the DHA, for instance, if the patient is registered with an NHS GP who is a fundholder or part of a fundholding consortium which was not party to the referral? At the time of writing, no clear answer to this question had been discovered.

References and further reading

Department of Health (1992) *The Statement of Fees and Allowances.* DoH, London.

Department of Social Security (1992) *Medical Evidence for Benefit Purposes.* DSS, London.

Department of Health and Social Security (1986) *Guide to the Management of Private Practice in Health Service Hospitals in England and Wales.* DHSS, London.

General Medical Council (1992) *Professional Conduct and Discipline: Fitness to Practise.* GMC, London.

Medical Ethics Committee, BMA (1992) *Rights and Responsibilities of Doctors.* BMA, London.

National Health Service (1992) *The NHS (General Medical Services) Regulations 1992. S.I.1992/635.* HMSO, London.

3

Consultant Practice and the NHS

Definitions

The Concise Oxford English Dictionary defines 'consultant' as a 'person consulted for professional advice, especially in a branch of medicine'. The NHS (Appointment of Consultants) Regulations prescribe who may enjoy this designation in the NHS, but there is no legal restriction as to who may use it in the private sector. The meaning of the term 'medical specialist' is similarly nebulous. In fact any qualified doctor can call himself a specialist, with or without the European Certificate of Specialist Training referred to earlier. In practice, however, the health insurers tend to confine specialist recognition to those who have at some time maintained a substantive consultant post in the NHS, a fact which has contributed a great deal to the recent public debate on the future of specialist training.

Relatively few specialists work exclusively and whole-time in the private sector (only 372 in 1992, according to BMA figures). The bulk of private practice is undertaken by consultants with an NHS contract. The records of insurance providers indicate that over 12 000 now undertake some private practice, if only the occasional out-patient consultation (and it has been estimated that there may be as many as 6000 retired NHS consultants in part-time private practice).

'Private practice' is defined for NHS consultants and other NHS hospital doctors (in paragraph 40 of the Terms and Conditions of Service of Hospital Medical and Dental Staff) as 'the diagnosis or treatment of patients by private arrangement'. This is said to include any general practice work carried out by consultants in general medical, dental or ophthalmic services. Private practice, so described, can be carried out under arrangements with health authorities in respect of in-patients or out-patients at NHS hospitals or entirely separately in private rooms or independent hospitals. A private patient is defined as a patient who has given an undertaking to pay (for accommodation and medical services).

Category 1 and category 2 work

Work involving diagnosis or treatment of NHS patients is known as category 1 work. This is to distinguish it from fee paid work which consultants are permitted to undertake in tandem with NHS work, which is known as category 2 work. Many people confuse private practice with category 2. In general, category 2 work does not involve treating patients. It may involve diagnosis, but for purposes other than those associated with treatment. The majority of such work involves examinations and reports for various non-NHS purposes, such as court proceedings, or to enable the patient to obtain social security or insurance benefits. An illustrative list of services which are regarded as category 2 work is provided in paragraph 37 of the Terms and Conditions of Hospital Medical and Dental Staff.

Where the consultant undertakes category 2 work and uses any of the hospital's radiological, technical or laboratory facilities, the terms and conditions of service oblige the consultant to pay one third of the fee he receives from the patient or third party to the hospital for the use of those facilities. Secretarial and administrative support are not included in the definition of technical facilities. The 'one third rule' does not apply, for complex historical reasons, to coroners' post-mortem examinations (*see* Chapter 16).

NHS consultant contracts (the '10% rule')

Private practice undertaken by whole-time consultants is subject to the 10% rule. In order to explain what this is it will first be necessary to explain the different types of NHS contract and their effect on consultants' ability to undertake private practice.

Consultants with whole-time or maximum part-time contracts work a minimum of 10 notional half days (NHDs), a NHD being defined as equivalent to 3½ hours 'worked flexibly'. They must both devote 'substantially the whole of their professional time' to NHS activities. However the whole-time contract holder is only allowed to undertake private practice provided it does not exceed 10% of his gross NHS earnings for a particular year (beginning 6 April). The maximum part-time contract holder, on the other hand, faces no restriction as to the amount he can earn from private practice. In return for this freedom the maximum part-timer is entitled to only 10/11 of the whole-timer's salary.

A part-time contract holder will have a work commitment of between one and nine NHDs. Part-timers are paid 1/11 of the whole-time consultants' salary for each NHD plus the same proportion of any distinction award held. However, unlike whole-timers or maximum part-timers, there is no contractual obligation on part-timers to devote substantially the whole of their professional time to the NHS (Table 3.1).

Whole-time contracts	— comprise a minimum of 10 NHDs
	— require the holder to devote substantially the whole of his professional time to the NHS
	— require that private practice income does not exceed 10% of gross NHS salary during two consecutive years
Maximum part-time contracts	— comprise a minimum of 10 NHDs but bring only 10/11 of the whole-timer's salary
	— require the holder to devote substantially the whole of his professional time to the NHS
	— involve no restriction on the amount of income from private practice
Part-time contracts	— comprise between 1 and 9 NHDs, each NHD = 1/11 of the whole-timer's salary
	— do not require substantial commitment of time to NHS
	— involve no restriction of private practice income

Table 3.1: NHS consultant contracts.

In 1991 there were about 10 500 full-time NHS consultants, 5000 maximum part-timers and 1500 part-timers. In addition there are estimated to be some 2200 honorary contract holders (*see* below). Apart from posts specifically defined as part-time, consultants have the option of commencing employment either as whole-timers or maximum part-timers. Because their contractual commitment to the NHS is identical, whole-timers can voluntarily change to maximum part-time contracts at any time, and maximum part-timers may revert to whole-time status, with the agreement of their employing authority, 'which may not unreasonably be withheld'. There is no question of consultants reducing their NHD commitment when they change from whole-time to maximum part-time or vice versa. However the 10% limit rules require compulsory regrading of whole-timers to maximum part-time status where the whole-timer has failed to bring his private earnings under control within the prescribed time span (*see* below).

Monitoring of compliance with the 10% rule

Whole-time consultants must certify annually to employing authorities at the end of the financial year that they have not exceeded the 10% limit. For the purposes of the 10% rule, gross NHS salary is taken to include any distinction award payable, but not other NHS emoluments such as fees for domiciliary visits. Authorities are entitled to call for the production of fully audited accounts to support certificates of earnings if necessary, though this is rarely exercised.

If a certificate is requested and not provided within three months, the employing authority may regard this as proof that private practice earnings are in excess of the 10% and take action accordingly. If consultants exceed the limit in two consecutive years from 6 April, and cannot show by the following 1 April that they have taken 'effective steps' to reduce their private commitments, they will automatically be regraded to a maximum part-time contract and lose 1/11 of their whole-time salary. They can only return to a whole-time status after a further two years in which their private earnings do not exceed the 10% limit.

Authorities cannot count part-years on a pro-rata basis. When consultants take up appointments on dates other than 6 April, authorities can only begin assessing compliance with the limit from the following 6 April. Deliberate repeated compliance only at the three-year stage is regarded as an abuse of the system. If a consultant knows in advance that his private earnings are likely to exceed the limit, and he has no intention of reducing them, he is advised to make this clear to his employers forthwith and seek to be regraded.

The BMA believes that consultants should act in accordance with the spirit of the rules governing the management of private practice at all times, fearing that non-compliance will bring the system into disrepute and result in greater restrictions being imposed. They remind consultants that any rights as to private practice, whether as whole-time or maximum part-time employees, do not allow them to diminish the level of service given to their NHS patients. They must give priority to their NHS work at all times, subject only to their ethical obligations to all their patients when emergencies arise.

'Substantial' commitment to the NHS

A National Audit Office (NAO) report on the NHS and the Independent Sector (HMSO 1989) raised the issue of monitoring and control of privately practising consultants' work commitments to the NHS, pointing out that there was no effective procedure in place for determining whether full-time consultants' private practice earnings remained below the 10% limit. The NAO found that no health authority they visited had any systematic mechanism for routine monitoring of compliance by consultants with their work programmes.

The report made reference to a study of private sector activity undertaken by the University of Sheffield Medical Care Research Unit in 1986 which indicated that, in aggregate, only 5% of the standard 10- or 11-session consultant working week in the main private practice specialties was not contracted to the NHS. The study found that during that limited time, or outside the standard working week, consultants performed one private in-patient operation for every seven that were performed (by themselves or their registrars) in the NHS, and one private day-case for every nine NHS day-cases. (A recent further study by Laing has confirmed that a considerable amount of private surgical activity in private hospitals takes place during unsocial hours, including weekends.)

While expressing disquiet over the absence of effective monitoring, the NAO concluded that the limited evidence available did not suggest significant neglect of NHS commitments by consultants generally. The Department of Health was nevertheless concerned to find a mechanism by which an individual's commitment could be regularly scrutinized. This was most effectively achieved by mandatory completion of work programmes or 'job plans'. Lengthy negotiations took place between the Department and the BMA culminating in the health circular, HC(90)16, which introduced this requirement for the first time in 1990.

While the DoH saw this as a means of regulating consultant activities and highlighting any abuses, the BMA saw this as a means of silencing critics who felt some consultants were neglecting their NHS duties, by showing just how great was the number of hours devoted on average to NHS activities. Recent estimates suggest that most whole-time and maximum part-time consultants work at least 50–60 hours per week (not counting time spent in on-call duties). Of this, the majority will devote less than 15% to private work. Since the promulgation of HC(90)16, concern on the part of the DoH at possible neglect of NHS duties by consultants seems largely to have abated.

Medical academics

There are about 2200 university medical school staff of NHS consultant status. The position of medical academics vis-à-vis private practice is rather complex. Clinical academic consultants may be employed under one of two possible types of contract:

1   an honorary contract, which is a contract with a medical or dental school or with the Medical Research Council, combined with an honorary (unpaid) appointment with a health authority

2   an A + B contract, under which the consultant may be employed: (a) on a part-time basis with both a medical or dental school or the Medical Research Council, and a health authority, or (b) jointly on a whole-time

basis with a medical or dental school or the Medical Research Council and/or health authority.

The ability of clinical academic staff to undertake private practice is affected by the nature of the contract under which they work. Consultants employed under the first option above are treated as part-timers by both the university and health authority and are not therefore subject to the 10% rule. Under the second option, consultants employed under (a) are considered to be part-timers and are therefore not normally subject to the 10% rule, whereas under (b) consultants will be looked upon as whole-time, and the 10% rule for private practice applies.

Generally speaking, universities place few restrictions on clinical academic staff undertaking private practice if the income is paid to the university. The right of honorary contract holders to undertake private practice for personal gain is a different matter and circumstances vary from university to university. Some permit personal gain from private practice on the same basis as NHS whole-time consultants, some prohibit paid employment outside the university contract, while others will allow honorary consultants to undertake private practice on the understanding that they retain only a proportion of the income, the remainder being paid to the institution. The Medical Academic Staff Committee of the BMA has argued for many years that clinical academic staff should be allowed to undertake private practice on the same basis as their NHS counterparts, and it continues to press the Committee of Vice Chancellors and Principals on this issue.

No figures are available about the amount of private practice that medical academics as a class are permitted to undertake. However, in the interim report of its Inquiry into private medical services, the MMC questions 'whether the arrangements under which consultants are obliged to surrender to the medical schools that employ them all or some of their earnings from private practice, restrict the supply of such services; with the result that charges generally for such services are higher than would be the case in the absence of those arrangements'. This would suggest that the amount of private practice undertaken by academics is significant.

One of the problems facing clinical academic staff undertaking private practice where remuneration is made over to their university is that they may still be liable for tax on fees earned in this context, even though they have derived no personal benefit from them. Any academic in this position would be well advised to seek advice from the university finance department and/or an accountant or the BMA regarding the status of payments made to the university.

Often fees derived from private practice are paid into departmental funds which are used for the purposes of education, eg paying for consultants to attend courses and symposia, or for the purchase of equipment. It is important to remember that the Inland Revenue will consider that the consultant who earned the fees in question is liable to pay tax on them except where an undertaking has been given to make over such remuneration into funds which are recognized by the tax authorities as having charitable status. The Inland Revenue may regard funds established for the educational purposes referred to above as having charitable status, particularly where the trust fund in question has been registered as a charity, but they may not necessarily do so. Medical academics should be wary of undertaking private practice until they have definitive advice from a tax expert on their specific circumstances in this connection.

The management of private practice in the NHS

Under the provisions of the NHS Act 1977 (or the NHS [Scotland] Act 1978), private patients could only be treated in NHS hospitals when the Secretary of State had authorized facilities to be used for this purpose. The NHS and Community Care Act 1990 amended this provision so that health authorities no longer need to seek such authorization. Health authorities are free to decide when and how many 'pay beds' are available to those staff who are entitled to admit their own patients to the hospital for NHS treatment. In almost all cases this will be to the hospitals' consultant staff only.

Pay beds are not beds exclusively set aside for private patients. When not occupied by private patients, they are used by NHS patients. There were about 3000 beds (in 850 hospitals) authorized for this purpose in 1991. Average occupancy by private patients was only about 32%. Health authorities may also offer patients 'amenity beds' for which a charge is made, or another category of private bed for which the patient pays but does not make any private arrangement for treatment with a consultant. In neither of these cases may the consultant charge any fees.

In accordance with the Health and Medicines Act 1988, health authorities are empowered to set their own charges for the cost of accommodation, equipment, drugs and the services of nursing and junior medical staff on what they consider to be the appropriate commercial basis (formerly, there was central guidance on the level of charges via NHS circulars). Consultants should therefore make themselves aware of the charging policy of the health authority where they work.

The *Guide to the Management of Private Practice in Health Service Hospitals in England and Wales* (The 'Green Book') was first published in March 1986 (December 1987 in Scotland). It was drawn up in consultation with representatives of the profession. One of its stated intentions was to ensure that the rules governing collection of income due to the NHS from private medical practice were properly applied. A revised version, taking account of changes brought about by the Health Service reforms contained in the NHS and Community Care Act 1990, was being prepared for issue in 1993/94.

All consultants should be in possession of the 'Green Book', and those who do not have a copy should request one from their employing health authority. The Green Book describes the procedure for authorizing pay beds, the application of charges, the practical aspects affecting income from private patients and, most importantly, the principles to be followed in conducting private practice in the NHS. These principles, generally referred to as the 'six principles' are as follows:

1 that the provision of services for private patients does not significantly prejudice non-paying patients

2 that, generally, early private consultations should not lead to earlier NHS admissions

3 that common waiting lists should be used for urgently and seriously ill patients

4 that, normally, access to diagnostic and treatment facilities should be governed by clinical considerations

5 that standards of clinical care and services should be the same for all patients

6 that single rooms should not be held vacant for potential private use longer than the usual time between NHS private admissions.

How private patients are received in NHS hospitals

The Green Book also details procedures for identifying private patients, and it is essential that consultants are aware of the procedures adopted in the hospital in which they work. The guidance stresses that it is the responsibility of consultants themselves to ensure that their private patients are identified as such. Hospitals are advised to establish mechanisms for identifying private referrals, the admission of private patients and the recovery of charges. Consultants using procedures agreed with management have a responsibility to identify to management in writing the status of any of their private in-patients or out-patients using NHS hospital facilities.

A private patient officer should be appointed at hospitals where private patients are treated. The private patient officer's job is to:

• provide information and advice to private patients on services and treatment

• ensure that the consultant and patient provide all necessary information for management and invoicing of costs

• ensure an undertaking to pay has been received

• ensure an appropriate deposit for costs of in-patient treatment is secured before admission

- ensure the patient is escorted to his accommodation on arrival and that the responsible clinician is informed accordingly

- ensure that adequate arrangements exist for all staff involved to identify all private patient activity which generate charges payable to the hospital

- monitor the number of private patient admissions.

The consultant with primary responsibility for the patient is responsible for telling the private patient officer when, in his clinical judgement, an episode of treatment is completed.

Change of status and other matters

It is important for consultants to be aware of the rules governing change of status by private patients. These were set out in the original Green Book as follows:

'22. *An out-patient cannot be both a private and an NHS patient for the treatment of one condition during a single visit to a health service hospital. A private out-patient at a NHS hospital is nonetheless legally entitled to change his status at a subsequent visit and seek treatment under the NHS ....*

23. *A private in-patient has a similar legal entitlement to change his status during the course of his stay in hospital. He might decide to exercise that entitlement when a significant and unforeseen change in circumstances arises, eg when he enters hospital for a minor operation and is found to be suffering from a different, more serious complaint. He remains liable to charges for the period during which he was a private patient ....*

24. *A change of status from private to NHS must be accompanied by an assessment of the patient's clinical priority for treatment as a NHS patient.*

25. *It is important that any private patient who wishes to become a NHS patient should gain no advantage over other NHS patients by so doing ....*

26. *Private patients who wish to revert to NHS status must therefore take the place appropriate to their clinical priority on the waiting list for hospital admission or for diagnostic procedures or for further in-patient treatment as appropriate. This rule must be applied, for example to private patients who see a consultant privately for an initial consultation—whether in the consultant's private consulting rooms, in the hospital or*

elsewhere—and who subsequently decide to become NHS patients, and health authorities will need to be able to identify such patients for monitoring purposes . . . .

27. A patient seen privately in rooms who then becomes a NHS patient joins the waiting list at the same point as if his consultation had taken place as a NHS patient. A consultant who has seen a patient privately in his rooms may, if he wishes, refer that patient to himself in his NHS clinic rather than referring the patient back to his GP.'

The Green Book also deals with the question whether common waiting-lists should include both urgent and seriously ill patients and those needing highly specialized diagnosis and treatment. It explains that, in accordance with the third of the six principles, private and NHS patients in these categories should be chosen for in-patient admission or out-patient attendance using the same criteria, irrespective of whether they are NHS or private patients.

Private patients from overseas should be dealt with in the same way as other private patients. Before admission they have to provide an undertaking to pay, and leave a deposit proportionate to the full estimated costs of the hospital charges. Hospitals generally seek full settlement of bills from such patients before they leave hospital.

The Green Book explains that the normal comprehensive pharmaceutical service in hospitals will be made available to resident private patients with full recovery of costs. In the case of private patients attending on an out-patient basis, the hospital doctor with clinical responsibility will also be responsible for prescribing any drug treatment. In such cases the prescription form FP10(HP) may not be used, but a private prescription may be written to be dispensed, unless it is a product restricted to hospital supply, either at the hospital pharmacy or in accordance with the patient's choice. Where the referring doctor (the GP) has accepted continuing responsibility or where there is an agreed 'shared care' arrangement, the hospital doctor may send the patient back to the referring doctor with the appropriate advice.

Involvement of other professionals

The hospital charges payable by private patients include an element for staff salaries other than those of consultants. Junior doctors are required as part of their normal duties under their terms and conditions of service to provide assistance, as directed by the consultant in charge, in managing the private patients under their care in an NHS hospital. They are not separately remunerated for this. They will normally only receive remuneration for assistance rendered to consultants in private hospitals, where such work is undertaken outside normal contracted hours.

Some consultants may wish to pay their junior colleagues for assisting them with private patients they treat in NHS hospitals. It should be remembered that in these circumstances the junior doctor will effectively be paid twice and their employing authority could argue that, by accepting payment for such assistance, they have invalidated the indemnity cover provided by the hospital, and would be personally liable for all 'acts and omissions' in the course of such treatment.

Associate specialists may treat the private patients of a consultant on a private basis only by special arrangement with the express agreement of that consultant in charge and the private patient.

When patients are admitted privately, the primary consultant should explain to the patient that the professional services of an anaesthetist and the opinion of a pathologist or radiologist may also be required and that fees will be payable for these services. Problems have arisen because of the practice of arranging the investigations of private patients through the NHS rather than privately. The BMA advises consultants to ensure that colleagues in the diagnostic specialties are properly involved in the treatment of private patients, and also encourages pathologists and radiologists to offer a personal service in return (*see* Chapter 16).

Contracts with third parties

Under section 7 of the Health and Medicines Act 1988, authorities can contract with third parties (eg private hospitals) to provide accommodation and services, as long as this does not significantly affect Health Service provision. These were formerly known as 'section 58' services (from the NHS Act 1977). A common example of this would be the provision of pathology services to a local private hospital. It is important to note that where a health authority proposes to provide such services, the agreement of the practitioners involved is required (in accordance with paragraph 31 of the Terms and Conditions of Service). The practitioners may negotiate separately with the third party to obtain fees for any of this work they undertake in this connection, which will be regarded as part of their normal gross income from private practice. Alternatively, by mutual consent, a sessional assessment may be made within the practitioner's NHS contract, and this work will not therefore be regarded as private practice.

Waiting-list initiatives

Following commencement of the NHS reforms, the Government sought to employ every possible means to reduce NHS waiting-lists. These waiting-list 'initiatives' included joint ventures with the private sector whereby health authorities agreed contracts for treatment of NHS waiting-list patients in private hospital facilities. In some cases the contract only covered the use of facilities, and treatment—which was undertaken by consultants in their NHS capacity—was paid for in the form of additional NHDs. In other cases, a health authority could purchase a whole package of facilities, including medical care, and the consultants undertaking the treatment received remuneration from the private hospitals. This work was clearly outside those consultants' NHS contracts, but the BMA's Central Consultants and Specialists Committee (CCSC) considered that it should not constitute private practice in the normal sense because it involved treatment of NHS patients which was paid for indirectly by the NHS.

Work for fundholders

They took a similar view of another development arising from the NHS reforms. This is the practice whereby GP fundholders are able to purchase the services of consultants by private arrangement, ie outside their contracts with NHS hospitals. A number of GP fundholders have contracted with consultants to undertake out-patient consultations either at the GP's surgery or in private rooms. This enables the fundholders' patients to be seen, and their need for further treatment to be diagnosed, more quickly (and frequently more cheaply) than via a contract with the hospital.

In discussing this with the Department of Health (DoH), the negotiating committee of the CCSC pointed out that, although such arrangements were 'private' insofar as the contracts were between the fundholders and individual consultants, the patients were NHS, not private patients, and their treatment was paid for by the NHS. They argued that this work, and that involved in the joint ventures referred to above, therefore constituted an entirely new category of fee paid work which they termed 'category 3'. The DoH refused to be swayed by these arguments and contended that, whatever the status of the patient and the source of funding, the 'private arrangement' in question was covered by the usual definition of private practice in paragraph 40 of the Terms and Conditions of Service and would therefore contribute towards the 10% limit of whole-time practitioners.

The CCSC issued advice to consultants accordingly, advising them to ensure that they obtain adequate medical indemnity cover for such work. Unfortunately the peculiar nature of the arrangements raises questions about the status of diagnostic tests (eg radiology and pathology) required as a result of such consultations (*see* Chapter 16).

Private practice and NHS Trust contracts

One of the potential benefits of self-governing Trust status for NHS hospitals is the ability to diverge from the national Terms and Conditions of Service for medical staff and to create new work-specific contracts and salary agreements. As part of the provisions of the NHS and Community Care Act 1990, consultants employed by hospitals becoming Trusts were 'transferred in' to those Trusts on their existing contracts and remained subject to the terms and conditions specified therein. Initially most Trusts were hesitant about offering substantially different contracts to newly appointed consultants, though they were free to do so.

However, new types of contracts are now being drawn up and accepted by new appointees. A distinguishing feature of many of these contracts is the imposition of conditions on the undertaking of private practice. Being always concerned with income generation, many Trusts are seeking to prohibit the undertaking of private practice by their employees other than within Trust facilities through which the Trust will derive a significant financial benefit. Some Trusts may go further and forbid their newly appointed consultants to retain any private fees, including category 2 fees. Others may require consultants to treat patients in the hospital's private facilities for no charge as part of their normal contractual requirements. Some Trusts are also seeking to tempt those on existing contracts to change to Trust contracts by offering to restore them to whole-time status and cancelling the 10% limit, for instance in return for loyalty clauses which require the consultants to bring all their private patients into Trust facilities.

The permutations of possible contractual arrangements within Trusts are endless, but it is clear that such developments will in time drastically alter the pattern of provision of private specialists' services, though it remains to be seen what the overall effect will be, both for specialists, patients, health insurers and private hospitals.

Reform of the system of specialist accreditation

As we have noted, the review of specialist accreditation undertaken by the working party chaired by the Department of Health's Chief Medical Officer, Dr Kenneth Calman, was prompted by concern at the discrepancy between the criteria for specialist accreditation adopted by the medical establishment in the UK and that applied elsewhere in the EC. This was initiated when the GMC decided to establish an indicative register of those who had 'completed' higher specialist training, with the suffix 'T' being shown after their names.

One of the principal stated purposes of the T register was to enable the public to distinguish those trained to consultant standards from those with less experience in the unregulated field of private practice. However, it was subsequently alleged that this system was discriminatory in respect of specialists from other European countries seeking to practise privately in the UK, and that it was unlawful in denying specialists having the European Certificate of Specialist Training (ECST) the equal status to which they are entitled as a consequence of the EC directives on mutual recognition of specialist training.

The Calman working party sought to resolve this dispute, while continuing to maintain the high standards required of consultants in the NHS: standards which incidentally the health insurers wished to see retained in the private sector. The debate subsequently crystallized into a conflict between, on the one hand, those who wanted to see the creation of a single specialist grade with less stringent requirements in terms of the period of training undertaken, and those who wished to preserve as far as possible the high standards guaranteed by the status quo.

The working party ultimately decided to recommend the reduction of the period of time necessary for completion of specialist training from an average of 10 to seven years and to make the award of the CCST the official hallmark of specialist status. As a result, thousands of senior registrars would, at a stroke become potentially eligible for consultant posts within the NHS.

What the representatives of the profession are now grappling with in discussions with the health departments is how the requisite number of new consultant posts can be created so as to provide jobs for these newly accredited specialists without abandoning altogether the principles given expression in the Department of Health document *Hospital Medical Staffing: Achieving a Balance*.

References and further reading

British Medical Association (1993) *Contractual Duties of Hospital Doctors: Categories 1 and 2*. (Guidance note).

Calman K (1993) *Hospital Doctors: Training for the Future—Report of the Working Group on Specialist Training*. DoH, London.

Central Consultants and Specialists Committee, BMA (1990) *Consultant's Guide for the '90s*. BMA, London.

Central Consultants and Specialists Committee, BMA (1990) *The Consultant Handbook*. BMA, London.

Department of Health and Social Security (1984) *Terms and Conditions of Service for Hospital Medical and Dental Staff*. DHSS, London.

Department of Health and Social Security (1986) *Guide to the Management of Private Practice in Health Service Hospitals in England and Wales*. DHSS, London.

Laing W (1993) *Laing's Review of Private Healthcare 1993*. Laing & Buisson, London.

Medical Ethics Committee, BMA (1992) *Rights and Responsibilities of Doctors*. BMA, London.

National Audit Office (1989) *The NHS and Independent Hospitals*. HMSO, London.

The NHS (Appointment of Consultants) Regulations 1982. S.I. 1982/276. HMSO, London.

UK Health Departments/Joint Consultants Committee/Chairmen of Regional Health Authorities (1986) *Hospital Medical Staffing: Achieving a Balance*. DoH, London.

4

Private Hospitals and Clinics

Private hospital groups in the UK

Prior to the advent of the NHS, most hospitals were private in sense of being independent and self-governing. There were at that time a number of 'municipal' as opposed to purely 'voluntary' hospitals, but it is probably true to say that there was a charitable element in the funding of all hospitals, dating back to medieval times and perhaps even before. The idea of the profit-making hospital is relatively modern, though it is rapidly increasing in importance in the UK, as its share of the amount of private treatment undertaken demonstrates. The revenue earned by non-profit-making or charitable hospitals in excess of operating costs is usually reinvested in the hospital or the group of which it is part.

In January 1993, according to an Independent Healthcare Association (IHA) survey, there were 221 independent hospitals with operating theatres in the UK, with a total of 11 306 beds for patients of all types. Since the mid-1980s there has been a resurgence in the development of new private acute units. By January 1993, 62% of beds were owned by 'for-profit' hospital operators, compared with only 41% in 1979. It has been estimated that the share of revenue controlled by these hospitals is substantially greater, at 69% for accounting periods ending in 1991.

A league table of independent hospital providers by numbers of hospitals and bed numbers, as of January 1993, is set out in Figure 4.1. The list is dominated by BUPA, the Compagnie Générale des Eaux (CGE) and Nuffield Hospitals, each with more than 1000 beds. In terms of operating revenue the CGE group topped the poll of providers in 1992–93, according to the Fitzhugh Directory, with BUPA in second place and Nuffield Hospitals third.

The fact that BUPA owns one of the largest groups of private hospitals goes some way towards explaining its continued dominance in the health insurance field. The merger between BUPA and the HCA group in the late 1980s resulted in an investigation by the Monopolies and Mergers Commission (MMC). In the event the MMC determined that their merger was not contrary to the public interest.

Operator	Hospitals	Beds
BUPA Health Services Ltd	29	1780
Compagnie Générale des Eaux (General Healthcare Group plc formerly AMI Healthcare Group plc & Great Northern Health Management Ltd exc. psych)	21	1657
Nuffield Hospitals	32	1297
Compass Healthcare Ltd	15	657
Community Hospitals Group plc	10	467
Independent British Hospitals Ltd	14	373
HCI Group plc	9	276
Wellington Private Hospital Ltd	1	267
St Martin's Hospitals Ltd	2	221
British Pregnancy Advisory Service	7	199
Paracelsus-Kliniken	3	175
Population Services FPP Ltd	4	85
Independent Care Management	2	84
Hospital Management Trust	2	60
Goldsborough Ltd	2	55
International Care Services	1	39
Nestor Medical Services Ltd	1	37

Table 4.1: Numbers of private hospitals and beds, 1993. (From Laing, 1993, based on data obtained from the Survey of Acute Hospitals in the Independent Sector, 1993.)

It has to be recognized that, by owning the hospitals in which a sizeable proportion of its subscribers are treated, BUPA is in a uniquely fortunate position among health insurers in being able to exercise direct control over hospital costs. The close links between BUPA and the Nuffield Hospital Group is another important factor. BUPA was instrumental in creating the Nuffield Group with the opening of the Wellington Humana Hospital in 1957 and, whatever the vicissitudes of this relationship since then, BUPA still enjoys a degree of influence with Nuffield Hospitals which other insurers might envy.

Some health insurers issue subscribers with lists of private hospitals which may, as in the case of BUPA, be graded in terms of cost and range of facilities as well as on geographical location. A full list of private hospitals and description of their facilities may be found in the Independent Healthcare Association Yearbook, the Fitzhugh Directory and Laing's Review of Private Healthcare.

Funding of private hospital activity

Private medical insurance (PMI) is the principal source of revenue for private hospitals, though other sources are probably more substantial than would be assumed. In 1993, Laing estimated that 70% of normally insurable private acute treatment was funded by PMI. This excluded 'fertility regulation' (ie family planning and abortion) and maternity and health screening, which are not covered by PMI policies. About 15% of private hospitals' income is generated by overseas patients. The remainder is made up of self-paying British patients.

The residue of independent hospital revenue is derived from contractual arrangements between the NHS and independent hospitals, though the majority of contracted beds used are in non-acute specialties including convalescence and terminal care. The NHS reforms have, as has been noted, given NHS purchasing authorities greater freedom to make use of the independent sector where it proves cost-effective, and there is a possibility of greater use in some areas in future. In fact the Conservative Government is keen to promote the idea of partnership between the NHS and the private sector and has sought to stimulate private investment in NHS facilities, even to the extent of inviting private companies to build and manage new NHS hospitals. However, the possible increase in use of NHS facilities for private patient care may have a deleterious effect on private hospitals, for whom the slightest downturn in bed occupancy rates could prove financially disastrous.

Health economists have noted that the rapid growth in private bed numbers in the 1980s, coupled with the increasing use of day surgery, has led to excess bed capacity in the private sector. The established private hospitals have occupancies around the mid-60% level; at less than 60% occupancy, profits are likely to be marginal. During 1990–92 the number of dedicated private patient units in the NHS increased from 25 to 80. Such units are likely to be highly competitive with the independent hospitals, since the average daily cost of acute in-patient care is considerably less in the NHS than in comparable private hospitals.

In terms of activity, a study by the Medical Care Research Unit of the University of Sheffield in 1986 found that 14.9% of elective surgery on residents of England and Wales was performed in independent hospitals (excluding contract beds). For some operations (eg hip replacements) and in some areas (eg the Home Counties) the proportion was substantially higher. Since then the expansion of PMI and increased claims rates suggests that in 1993 the figure may be as high as 20–25%. However, abortion remains the most common procedure carried out in independent hospitals. Of the total of 180 000 legal abortions carried out in England and Wales in 1991, 104 000 were in the independent sector.

Relationship with consultants

Apart from in certain clinics and psychiatric hospitals, medical practitioners working in private hospitals do so as independent contractors, not as salaried employees. They are granted the privilege of being able to admit patients, subject to specified conditions and to be solely responsible for the patient's care during their stay in hospital.

This means that hospitals rely on the consultants to whom they have granted admission rights to bring in the patients on whom their business depends. There is therefore sometimes a degree of competition between private hospitals in some areas, with each seeking to obtain the allegiance of local specialists by offering high-quality facilities and equipment, and competent and efficient staff. Hospitals will also seek to draw their services to the attention of local GPs who, by referring patients to consultants associated with that hospital, will improve the level of business activity.

'Cost ratings' for health insurance

However, for a private hospital to enjoy any business at all, it must secure recognition by the private health insurers. The insurers publish lists of hospitals banded according to price, with admission to the most expensive (often in London) being restricted to subscribers with the most expensive policies. Hospitals therefore have a vested interest in keeping their costs down, as the lower the cost rating attributed to them, the greater will be the number of insured patients they can expect to attract. Price competition between hospitals is also particularly important in attracting non-insured patients, who will be more anxious to shop around as they will have to meet the full costs themselves.

Private hospital charges

Private acute hospitals often publish details of standard charges for accommodation and the use of operating theatres. In practice, rates may differ from those published, and they will not in any case include drugs and dressings, which are charged for separately. The majority of private hospitals are now offering 'package deals' involving fixed-price surgery for specific types of operation, usually intended for non-insured patients. Such contracts may involve an element covering the consultant's fees which may be lower than what the specialist would normally charge for his services in order to generate additional demand.

Regulation and management of private hospitals

Registration and inspection of private hospitals and nursing homes is carried out by health authorities under the aegis of the Registered Nursing Homes Act 1984. The scope of this legislation is broadly permissive. For practical purposes private hospital development is subject only to local authority planning controls. Prior to 1990 the Secretary of State for Health had to receive and authorize all applications within the scope of the Health Services Act 1980. This excluded non-surgical facilities as well as units with fewer than 120 beds and expansions which would add less than 20% of the total bed complement in any health district in any three-year period. The NHS and Community Care Act 1990 eliminated most of the remaining central government restrictions on development activity.

Interestingly, the provisions of the 1984 Act apply wholly to the regulation of premises and equipment by means of inspection and registration by health authorities. They do not prescribe any standards as regards personnel and the competence of medical practitioners who may be employed. The regulations refer only to the obligation to provide 'adequate professional, technical, ancillary and other staff' and 'adequate medical, surgical and nursing equipment and adequate treatment facilities'.

The particulars required to be furnished by an applicant for registration include 'the full names and qualifications of any resident or non-resident employed medical practitioner'. The health authority could refuse to register a private hospital if such particulars were not provided, but its powers to influence the choice of practitioner and thereby the standard of treatment offered are negligible. The Secretary of State does have power to regulate certain types of treatment, eg abortion, but there is at present no central means of assessing standards or accrediting private institutions. In this regard the private sector is entirely self-regulating.

Admission rights

Arrangements governing admission rights to private hospitals are therefore the subject of an agreement between the consultant and hospital concerned. These arrangements are not always the subject of a written contract, though standard contracts have been developed for use in some of the larger private hospital groups. It may be useful to detail the particulars contained in such contracts, (which are, for the most part, consistent with those of the unwritten variety).

The 'rights granted' often comprise the right to:

- admit patients to beds in the hospital
- utilize the facilities of the operating theatre and treatment rooms
- make arrangements for provision of anaesthetics (sometimes only by anaesthetists specifically approved by the hospital)
- prescribe drugs, and order X-rays, pathology and other laboratory services, physiotherapy and any other available facilities incidental to treatment of the patients under the practitioner's supervision
- use consulting rooms in the hospital (subject to terms agreed for the time being).

The private hospital will usually require the practitioner to manage matters such as obtaining appropriate informed consent to treatment from the patient. For legal reasons the hospital will not wish to involve its directly employed staff in such matters. The hospital will also insist on proof of the practitioner being fully registered with the GMC and being a fully paid-up member of one of the medical defence organizations. A standard written contract usually requires the practitioner to notify the hospital of any matter which adversely affects either his registration or defence society subscription.

Termination of admission rights

Apart from ceasing to be registered with the GMC, or allowing defence society subscriptions to lapse, most private hospitals provide for routine termination of admission rights for practitioners reaching the age of 70, though a moratorium can be granted exceptionally. Acrimonious disputes have occasionally arisen as a result of a provision in the standard contract of one of the larger hospital groups to terminate admission rights at the end of a defined period of notice (eg three months) without assigning a reason. Unfortunately there is no obvious legal remedy should this situation occur, provided it is written into the standard agreement on admitting rights. Fortunately terminations of admitting rights on such grounds are extremely rare.

Management of patients in private hospitals

The private hospital manager is understood to be in overall administrative control of all hospital departments and staff. Day-to-day control of nursing staff is vested in the matron who, curiously, occupies in the private hospital an elevated position similar to that which the matron used to enjoy in NHS hospitals. However it is important to recognize that the practitioner (consultant) has overall clinical responsibility for the patients he has admitted, subject to the arrangements agreed. The practitioner acts as an intermediary between the patient and the hospital. The hospital is indemnified against the effects of any professional failings on his part but is free to levy charges for use of facilities arranged by the practitioner directly of the patient without his involvement.

Although the influence of the Medical Advisory Committee (*see* below) is not to be underestimated, the clinical autonomy of consultants with admission rights in private hospitals is vouchsafed to an equal, if not greater, degree than in the NHS. Once again the private sector is a slightly distorted reflection of the image of practice prevailing in the public sector.

The practical arrangements for managing the patient during his stay are as follows. The practitioner is usually required to provide the hospital with written information concerning his patient prior to admission. This might include a statement of the patient's current problem and condition, relevant past medical history, current medication and any known allergies. The practitioner may also be required to deposit his case notes (or a photocopy) with the hospital during the patient's stay. These will be updated and returned to the practitioner when treatment has been completed. A discharge summary should also be despatched to the patient's GP.

Some hospitals offer assistance to practitioners in the way of collecting professional fees from the patient, but they will disclaim responsibility for collecting fees other than via the locally agreed scheme.

Choice of private hospital

The choice of hospital at which a newly appointed consultant will seek admitting rights will be determined largely by its location in terms of proximity to the NHS hospital where the consultant works or to his home. He will not wish to accept responsibility for patients who cannot be reached within a reasonably short time. It may also be influenced by the standard of facilities the hospital has to offer the consultant and his patients. In looking round a private hospital it may be appropriate to give particular attention to the quality of paramedical departments such as pathology, radiology, physiotherapy and pharmacy. Where these are not provided on site it can lead to complications, and the practitioner is advised to enquire about arrangements for these services.

Practitioners' financial interests

Apart from money paid specifically for the rent or lease of consulting rooms within the hospital confines, practitioners do not pay private hospitals any consideration for the privilege of admitting patients to their facilities. Nor should the hospital pay any consideration to the practitioner in return. This is expressly forbidden by the strict rules laid down by the GMC regarding such matters. The GMC is of course concerned to ensure that doctors base any decision about where to refer or admit a patient solely on the best interests of the patient's treatment. It therefore advises doctors to disclose any financial interest they might have in a private hospital or nursing home before referring the patient to any such institution. The pronouncements of the GMC in its document *Professional Conduct and Discipline: Fitness to Practice* (the 'Blue Book') on this subject are worth quoting in full:

'115. *A doctor who recommends that a patient should attend at, or be admitted to, any private hospital, nursing home or similar institution, whether for treatment by that doctor or by another person, must do so only in such a way as will best serve, and will be seen best to serve, the medical interests of the patient. Doctors should therefore avoid accepting any financial or other inducement from such an institution which might compromise, or be regarded by others as likely to compromise, the independent exercise of their professional judgment. Where doctors have a financial interest in an organisation to which they propose to refer a patient for admission or treatment, whether by reason of a capital investment or a remunerative position, they should always disclose that they have such an interest before making the referral.*

116. *The seeking or acceptance by a doctor from such an institution of any inducement for the referral of patients to the institution, such as free or subsidised consulting premises or secretarial assistance, may be regarded as improper. Similarly, the offering of*

such inducements to colleagues by doctors who manage or direct such institutions may be regarded as improper.'

Notwithstanding these pronouncements, consultants who have consulting rooms in a particular private hospital may well feel that it would benefit the patients who they see there and who require in-patient treatment to admit them to that same hospital where they are based.

Medical Advisory Committees

Most private hospitals have a Medical Advisory Committee (MAC) which hospital management will consult on all medical matters affecting the hospital, particularly new requests for admitting rights. (This should not be confused with the Hospital Medical Society which exists for purely social functions associated with the hospital.)

The constitution of MACs may vary but it will usually comprise representatives of all the main specialties (between 10 or 12 individuals), together with the hospital manager and matron, but it is customary for it to be able to co-opt additional specialists and hospital staff as and when required. The principal functions of the MAC are to advise the hospital management on the following matters:

- the granting or termination of admitting rights
- deficiencies or improvements needed in hospital facilities (including employed staff)
- whether and how new forms of treatment available in particular specialties can be accommodated
- clinical matters affecting practice, including on rare occasions matters involving the behaviour of individual consultants.

Just as the health insurers regard an NHS consultant appointment as the principal criterion for the purposes of specialist recognition, private hospitals, advised by their MACs, invariably follow the same line. Indeed it is difficult to see how they could do otherwise, bearing in mind the health insurers' rules on reimbursement, since admission of patients by specialists not recognized by health insurers could prejudice reimbursement of the hospital costs by the insurer. Occasionally the MAC may decide to accord admitting rights to non-specialists (ie GPs) in the specific context of psychiatric or geriatric medicine, allowing them a limited number of beds to which to admit long-stay patients requiring mainly nursing care. However the absence of health insurance reimbursement is a considerable disincentive to such proposals.

The main purpose of the MAC is to advise on clinical matters, but it also serves as a forum in which the users of the facilities can air grievances and discuss developments or potential developments affecting their practice in the hospital.

The role of the MAC chairman is pivotal in relations between consultants using the hospital and the hospital management. The chairman is elected either by the MAC or directly by all the consulting users, but in practice he must be an individual in whom both management and professional colleagues have complete confidence. Appointment as chairman of the MAC is therefore considered to be a mark of some esteem. Occasionally the chairmen of MACs of different hospitals within the same hospital group will meet together to discuss developments of common interest and meet representatives of the insurers and other bodies. By this means they can wield considerable influence on the functioning of the private health sector and relay useful information back to the MAC.

Recently the role of MACs has been criticized to some extent, in a report sponsored by Norwich Union Healthcare, by an organization calling itself National Economic Research Associates (NERA). The report notes that in normal circumstances the ability of existing suppliers of a service to control entry would be regarded with suspicion. It admits that in practice MACs normally grant admission rights to newly qualified NHS consultants without question, but declares that there is less clarity about applications from time-expired senior registrars, foreign doctors and established consultants attempting to expand their private practice into neighbouring areas. NERA therefore concludes that 'the rules of MACs require some scrutiny to ensure that appropriately qualified medical practitioners are not denied access to private hospitals in order to protect the interests of incumbents'.

Audit and peer review

Medical audit is an inescapable feature of practice in the post-reform NHS. It is also beginning to have an impact on the private sector. While it is not always possible to compare NHS and private practice, the health insurers are keen to use audit as a means of improving quality. It is certainly a bonus point in any public relations activity. The private hospitals are taking a lead in this regard by drawing up codes of good practice. The BUPA hospitals have produced one such guide which distinguishes between the work expected of the clinician in charge and that of other hospital staff, and which stresses the need for adequate records, operation notes and discharge summaries.

MACs are helping to improve the quality of service in the private sector by means of peer review. In some hospitals panels of volunteer representatives from each specialty have been appointed, entrusted with the task of implementing protocols for audit and clinical standards.

One of the concerns which private hospitals have is to ensure that they are not out of step with the development of good practice in the NHS. If the private hospitals are to compete with NHS Trust hospitals and directly managed units for the contracts offered by district health authorities and fundholders, they will have to be able to demonstrate a commitment to maintain clinical standards equal to, if not surpassing, those of the NHS.

The data derived from audit may also serve the interests of the health insurers in other ways. The insurers have become concerned at the way in which certain conditions which are no longer fashionable in the NHS, like tonsillectomy or removal of wisdom teeth, continue to represent a major proportion of operations undergone in the private sector, (indeed extraction of wisdom teeth is generally reckoned to be the most commonly performed private operation). There is certainly a feeling among many insurers that a lot of unnecessary surgery may be taking place in the private sector judging by the extent to which treatment of such conditions involving surgery has diminished in the NHS. The data from such activities will undoubtedly assist the health insurers in their efforts to contain costs by regulating the scope of private practitioners' activities (*see* Chapters 5 and 6).

References and further reading

Blair P and National Economic Research Associates (1993) *Healthcare Report: Reforming the Private Sector*. Norwich Union Healthcare, Norwich.

British United Provident Association (1992) *A Guide to Private Consultant Practice*. BUPA, London.

General Medical Council (1992) *Professional Conduct and Discipline: Fitness to Practice*. GMC, London.

Healthcare Information Services (1992) *The Fitzhugh Directory of Independent Healthcare Financial Information 1992–93*.

Independent Healthcare Association (1993) *The Directory of Independent Hospitals and Health Services*. Longman, London.

Laing W (1993) *Laing's Review of Private Healthcare*. Laing & Buisson, London.

Monopolies and Mergers Commission (1990) *The British United Provident Association Ltd and HCA UK Ltd: A Report on the Merger Situation*. HMSO, London.

Office of Health Economics (1992) *Compendium of Health Statistics 1992*. HMSO, London.

The Registered Nursing Homes and Mental Nursing Homes Regulations 1984. S.I.1984/1578. HMSO, London.

5

Private Medical Insurance

The nature of the health insurance market

Approximately 12% of the UK population (about 7 million people) are covered by some form of private medical insurance. This accounts for approximately 70% of private hospital treatment. For many doctors, particularly those of the older generation, health insurance is synonymous with the provident associations. This is the term used to describe the three largest health insurers, the British United Provident Association (BUPA), Private Patients Plan (PPP) and the Western Provident Association (WPA), and a number of smaller organizations (*see* Appendix).

A provident association is a non-profit-making organization, rather like a mutual insurance company. That is to say, any revenue it enjoys, in excess of its operating costs, becomes part of the company's reserves which have to be reinvested in facilities or services which are of direct benefit to its subscribers (and are not therefore subject to corporation tax). It is registered with the Department of Trade and Industry as an insurance company limited by guarantee but does not have shareholders, except where its subscribers are considered to be its shareholders. It is not exactly a charity, though the objective of its activity is to benefit the totality of its subscribers.

The providents were set up specifically to facilitate health insurance, their intention being to enable subscribers to fund treatment they might not otherwise be able to afford all at once. To the outsider, of course, there may be no discernible difference between a provident association and a profit-making insurance company. They act like large corporate institutions. They market their policies like any other insurer and also no more likely to act beneficently towards their subscribers. The cynic might argue that using revenue to purchase private hospitals or foreign insurance companies is not a direct benefit to subscribers and is really no more than a convenient means of absorbing profits in capital ventures.

In fact some of the provident associations show signs of a certain schizophrenia in relation to the business they are in. The provident with the largest market share, BUPA, is not a member of the Association of British Insurers

(ABI), for instance, presumably believing that its status is not that of a health insurer per se. On the other hand the PPP group, the second largest provident, is a member of the General Insurance Council of the ABI.

The fact that the market in PMI continues to be dominated by the provident associations encourages the continued use of the term 'provident' as shorthand for 'private health insurer'. However, the market share of the big three providents, BUPA, PPP and WPA, is no longer sacrosanct. Their collective market share has been gradually declining, from 91% in 1985 to 83% in 1991. One reason for this is the move into PMI by 'commercials' including some very large mainstream insurance companies like Norwich Union and Sun Alliance. These companies are intent on carving out a sizeable share of the market for themselves and their ability to do so, or to create new markets for individual and corporate health insurance by means of cheap and innovative policies, should not be underestimated.

The dominance of the health insurance market by BUPA was for many years unchallenged, though in recent years its share has been eroded by rivals, principally PPP, and some of the new players in the marketplace. A series of financial problems not directly related to the health insurance business has contributed to its apparent decline from over 60% in 1989 to 49% of the market in 1991 (Fig 5.1). BUPA is nevertheless still very much *the* health insurer as far as the public are concerned. In terms of brand-name recognition, rival companies hardly feature in consumer studies.

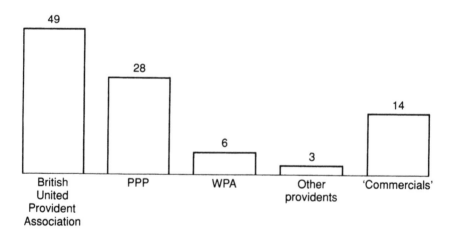

Figure 5.1: The market in private health insurance. PMI market share by subscription income 1991. (From Laing and Buisson, 1992.)

The structure of the health insurance business is an important consideration for all concerned with it, including its 'providers'. A survey of the big three providents undertaken in 1988 showed that 57% of their business was made up of corporate schemes, 15% of group schemes and 27% of individual subscribers. (Group schemes involve members of association groups, like credit-card holders and members of motoring organizations, and trade and professional bodies, for whom a modest group discount is allowed.)

Health insurance cover for employees has become part of the standard package of perks with which large firms attempt to recruit and retain valued staff. In the recession of the early 1990s, however, many companies began to find this an expensive luxury. The desire to minimize costs has led to a good deal of business being transferred from one insurer to another, often on advice from brokers. It has also led to the proliferation of a new concept, that of self-insurance, whereby company employees are invited to contribute directly into funds set up by their employers who manage and administer their own scheme or use the services of health insurers only to a limited extent. The development of this concept has been impeded to a certain extent, however, by taxation difficulties.

Relationship with 'providers'

So much for the business: but how does the operation of the health insurance market affect doctors in private practice? As has been noted earlier, the provident associations had not, until recently, sought to interfere in the way the patient and his GP chose and established a contract with an individual specialist. It was accepted that the contract between the insured patient and the doctor on the one hand, and between the insured patient and the health insurer on the other, were mutually distinct. The relationship between insurers and individual providers of private health care was therefore indirect.

However, for various reasons the insurers have recently sought to influence the choice of specialist. One reason for this is a concern to guarantee quality, apparently in order to maintain public confidence in private healthcare. The other is a desire to contain the increasing cost of private healthcare. Both of these reasons may be sublimated to a single broad objective: a desire to exercise greater control over their business environment. The insurers are no longer content to leave such an important aspect of their business to its own devices: to grow organically, so to speak. Insurers need to anticipate how their money is being spent, and are concerned to channel its direction to a far greater extent than heretofore.

Specialist recognition

The attempt to guarantee quality has been undertaken principally by means of the establishment of strict criteria governing the type of specialist in respect of whose treatment costs will be reimbursed to the insured. The rules of many health insurance policies stipulate that treatment must be provided by an approved specialist and that, to be approved, the specialist must have held a substantive NHS consultant post or be accredited by one of the Royal Colleges or Joint Committees for Higher Specialist Training. Many specialists who, for one reason or another, left the NHS before obtaining a substantive NHS consultant post have been adversely affected by this, and a great many doctors active in sub-specialties which do not have their own faculty or other means of specialist accreditation (eg orthopaedic physicians) have found their freedom to treat insured patients impeded to a great extent.

Unfortunately the insurers have not always adopted a consistent approach. Some allow themselves a considerable measure of flexibility as regards the recognition of those whom they regard as being of equivalent status, and because such decisions are made in secret, this has led to a good deal of criticism among practitioners affected.

Now that the Calman report (*see* Chapter 3) has forced the UK government to countenance a change in the procedures for recognizing the completion of specialist training, it remains to be seen whether the health insurers will continue to be wedded to what the establishment prescribes, or whether—in a continued attempt to maintain the highest standards—they will be tempted to 'move the goalposts' and devise some alternative or additional criteria in order to exclude those specialists whom they had not previously accredited.

Age limit on specialists

The restrictions inherent in the health insurers' criteria for specialist recognition were taken a step further by BUPA when, as of January 1992, it introduced an amendment to the rules of all its schemes, confining recognition to specialists under 70 years of age. As we have seen, most private hospitals already insist on termination of admitting rights when the practitioner reaches 70 years of age. Only in rare circumstances are consultants in the NHS permitted to continue beyond the normal NHS retirement age of 65. BUPA justified its decision in terms of public interest and concern 'to maintain public confidence in private health care'.

Many practitioners objected to this 'age discrimination'. There was general agreement that it was inappropriate for consultants to undertake major surgery beyond the age of 70, but it was pointed out that there were many eminent physicians and psychiatrists, for instance, whose services were in demand by patients and GPs, who would no longer be able to treat BUPA subscribers. The failure of the majority of the specialist fraternity to support the protests of the minority of senior colleagues affected put paid to any chances of a climbdown by BUPA, although the adverse publicity may well have dissuaded PPP, which had expressed an intention to follow suit, from taking up this proposal.

Exclusions from health insurance

We have noted that private health insurance has generally been confined to 'the cure and relief' of *acute* conditions. Recognizing that treatment of *chronic* conditions (such as renal dialysis) and palliative care (such as hospice treatment of the terminally ill) were ruinously expensive, the insurers made virtually no provision for such treatment. The insurers have also for many years either excluded or placed restrictions on treatment of drug or alcohol dependence. Recently the desire to contain costs has led them to institute further exclusions and stricter rules governing existing treatments which are likely to be of long duration, particularly psychiatric treatment.*

Most insurers currently place a limit on the number of days of in-patient psychiatric treatment for which benefit is payable, but as from 1992 BUPA has insisted on prior authorization by them of in-patient admissions for psychiatric treatment, while PPP requires either pre-authorization or 'utilization review' (*see* Chapter 16).

Cost containment measures

The health insurers are now considering a wide range of options aimed at reducing costs generally, including the cost of professional fees. Chief among these is the idea of establishing clinical protocols. There have been moves in the NHS to try and minimize unnecessary expenditure by developing such protocols, against which the activities of individual consultants or departments can be judged. These involve detailed research, out of which representative panels of learned clinicians deduce a consensus of opinion governing a particular procedure. This might concern, for instance, the length of in-patient stay following such an operation. From the available data, an 'average' would be established and a protocol drawn up covering situations during which an earlier or later date of discharge might be justified. The larger health insurers have been actively courting the Royal Colleges and individual experts in an attempt to establish such protocols for the more expensive areas of consultant activity. Publication of these protocols provides the insurers with the means with which to query 'excessive' charges by clinicians or hospitals. By doing so they may restrict further the clinical freedoms of individual con-

---

* A study by the Wyatt company in 1992 revealed that 40% of its sample companies excluded psychiatric illness from their group schemes and nearly 73% excluded alcoholism/drug dependence.

sultants, though it could be argued that these are already being restricted to the same extent in the NHS.

Yet another cost-containment measure borrowed from the NHS is the encouragement given to day-case surgery. BUPA has again taken the lead in this by establishing greater facilities for day-case surgery and actively encouraging their use by offering a 10% supplement on the standard price of an operation where it is undertaken on a day-case basis. Some have queried whether such incentives might lead to inappropriate use of the day-case option and therefore constitute an encouragement to unethical behaviour. A statement by the company suggested that the proportion of day-case surgery undertaken in its hospitals had increased to 40% by 1992.

Direct settlement

Another means of controlling the business environment is by means of the direct settlement of bills. The insurers had little leverage with private hospitals when payments were made to the insured person to pass on to the treatment providers. By agreeing to settle bills directly, the insurers were able to exercise greater control over the costs of both hospitals and specialists. Through direct settlement, insurers are able to query excessive charges. They can also exploit the more direct contacts established in order to persuade hospitals to offer more competitive prices. The attempt to contain hospital costs has not been universally successful, however. While the insurers have concentrated on bringing down the price of in-patient stays there is, according to *Laing's Review*, some evidence that the private hospitals have simply responded by shifting charges onto ancillary items such as drugs and diagnostic services.

By offering to pay consultants directly, the insurers have also been able to query excessive professional fees. The medical directors or advisers of the larger insurers now routinely correspond with consultants about charges for individual subscribers and, using entreaty, cajolement or (in the last resort) warnings that the consultant may incur a permanently adverse reputation with the insurer concerned, are often able to persuade practitioners to reduce their bills. Direct settlement may seem a more practical arrangement for practitioners at first glance, but it is not without its problems (*see* Chapter 13).

Managed care

All of these cost-containment measures may be regarded as part of an overall strategy aimed at reducing claims costs, known as 'managed care'. This concept emerged in the USA in the second half of the 1980s as a means by which corporations aimed to counter inflation of medical care costs. The elements of managed care developed in the USA are as follows:

- prior review of appropriateness of care (pre-authorization)
- encouragement of day-case surgery
- review of preoperative stay
- review of length of stay
- restriction of access to efficient suppliers
- prevention and control of catastrophic (exorbitant) care costs
- programmes designed to promote healthy lifestyle or 'wellness'
- centres of excellence to undertake high-cost therapies efficiently.

The advocates of managed care usually cite two possible approaches: one, described as the 'velvet glove' approach, involves pre-claims counselling of subscribers and persuading clinicians to move closer to 'best practice' through peer pressure and by providing information about this in the form of clinical protocols; the other is 'full-blown' managed care, characterized by pre-authorization of claims, nomination of hospital of treatment and reimbursement limited to a specified length of stay. As we have seen, both approaches are being used in the case of psychiatric treatment and may, in due course, be extended to other areas.

Control of professional fees

Yet there is a further and much more effective means of controlling the levels of professional fees. For several years BUPA maintained a schedule of individual operations, broken down into five basic categories: minor, intermediate, major, major plus and complex. Originally this schedule was unpublished, although BUPA made available to practitioners and subscribers the benefit levels appropriate to the different categories. Given the predominance of BUPA, these levels of reimbursement effectively became the 'industry standard'. PPP produced a similar schedule but provided no information about the 'reasonable' levels beyond which reimbursement would not be made. In the absence of any other published limits, the other health insurers came to regard the BUPA categories as an index of the 'going rate' for specialist fees. Whilst a consultant was theoretically free to charge what he thought reasonable, the limit of reimbursement was and is a significant constraint. Consultants do not relish the prospect of haggling with their patients over shortfalls between the bills submitted and the amount reimbursed to the patient, and were therefore given a considerable incentive to set their fees in accordance with BUPA benefit levels.

The amounts allowed by BUPA for professional fees were, moreover, a composite of amounts allowed for both surgeon and anaesthetist. In general it was assumed that the proportion of surgeons' to anaesthetists' fees would be in the order of 2:1. However it soon became clear that a great many privately practising consultants were becoming restive at the 'straitjacket' imposed by the BUPA categories.

The level and frequency of increases in these rates very soon became a major source of friction between BUPA and the profession's representatives. Some members of the profession resented what they saw as 'downward pressure' being exerted on professional fees in what was supposed to be a free market for services. Discussions took place between BUPA and the BMA, but when these failed to bring about any significant movement towards the improvements it considered necessary, the BMA responded by producing its own alternative fees for private operations.

The BMA Guidelines

The document entitled *Private Consultant Work: BMA Guidelines* was first published in 1989. This was a detailed fee schedule based on data obtained from the three major provident associations. However the principal difference between the BMA Guidelines and the BUPA schedule was that the former offered a specific guideline figure for each operation rather than confining itself to broad categories. It also differentiated between surgeons' and anaesthetists' fees and established the relative values of each on the contribution made in the context of that specific operation. They thus abandoned the old 2:1 ratio, adjudging each procedure on its merits.

The publication of the BMA Guidelines may have prompted BUPA to make its schedule publicly available to its providers, which it did for the first time in 1990, having subdivided the five categories so that there were henceforward 25 categories of operation.

A further change which may owe much to the example set by the Guidelines was the introduction by BUPA in 1991 of a separate scale of fees for anaesthetists. This required a substantial extra cash injection, as BUPA could not justify a diminution in the fees for surgeons, in order to reward anaesthetists more fairly. It was able to offset these costs, however, by making savings elsewhere, for instance by declaring a number of procedures to be eligible for only a 'minor addition' to the fee for an out-patient consultation.

Many of BUPA's rivals appear to have found the BMA Guidelines a valuable tool in determining a reasonable level of fee to reimburse for particular operations. However, the reception given to the BMA schedule by the health insurers generally began to change over time as the BMA sought, as in 1991, to increase the relative values it had established to be the 'average' charge, by an amount equal to that by which consultants' NHS remuneration was increased, on the recommendations of the Doctors' and Dentists' Review Body (DDRB). The fact that two successive DDRB awards exceeded the retail price index was not lost on the health insurers, some of whom began to complain openly about 'inflationary tendencies'.

However the BMA's right to publish its schedule went unchallenged until the Office of Fair Trading (OFT) decided to investigate the possible effects of the publication on the market in private healthcare. Following a brief investigation in early 1992 the OFT referred the question of fees for private medical services to the Monopolies and Mergers Commission in July of that year (*see* Chapter 6).

Medical inflation: competition and claims incidence

Through all this, the stated aim of all health insurers has been to contain costs. Medical inflation is clearly a matter of grave concern, but just how justified is this concern? Is the revenue from PMI diminishing in relation to expenditure? Some experts have speculated that the major insurers have always wanted to maintain a high-priced service so as to maintain its perceived value as a status-related fringe benefit. Research by the Centre for Health Economics at the University of York published in 1990, indicated that demand for health insurance was relatively insensitive to its price. This theory is supported by the private healthcare economist William Laing, who has consistently maintained the view that demand for PMI is 'price inelastic'. In other words, a decrease in the cost of premiums will not lead to a corresponding increase in the number of subscribers. However it is clear that many of the new commercial insurers wish to see an expansion of the PMI market and are leading the way in offering cheap policies which are proving to be attractive to individual subscribers at the lower end of the market. The larger health insurers have had to respond to this by introducing similar policies of their own (eg BUPA's 'Healthchoice' and the PPP's 'Value plan').

Competition, particularly from the arrival of new companies with a mainstream insurance background, has undoubtedly put pressure on the major insurers to reduce the cost of subscriptions and attract new customers. Competition is therefore putting the squeeze on profits as much as if not more so than medical inflation. This is compounded by another significant factor, namely the overall increase in the number of claims made by subscribers. For reasons which are not altogether clear, subscribers are making more use of their policies than in the past so that, while keeping subscriptions low to maintain market share and thereby reducing revenue, the insurers are having to pay out more in benefits. As *Laing's Review* (1993) explains: 'It is widely recognised among insurers . . . that increased claims frequency is the main reason why PMI cost inflation has run ahead of RPI.' During 1991 the average of benefits as a percentage of subscription revenue stood at a record 88%. The insurers were forced to increase subscription levels markedly in order to restore profitability.

To survive in this type of business environment the insurers are more anxious than ever to contain costs. However, the medical profession may be forgiven for feeling that they are being made the scapegoat for faults inherent in the system of private healthcare provision. There is certainly no evidence to suggest that medical fees are increasing at a greater rate than hospital costs, for instance. The proportion of costs attributable to medical fees has remained remarkably constant during the last 20 years at around one third of the total. There is, nevertheless, a very strong feeling among health insurers (given expression in the Laing/Norwich Union report—*see* Chapter 6) that private medical fees are probably 'substantially higher than necessary to ensure the availability of an appropriate level and range of specialist skills'. This has led some of them to consider for the first time the possibility of reducing professional fees by means of changes to the system of private healthcare provision.

References and further reading

British Medical Association (1992) *Private Consultant Work: BMA Guidelines 1992.* BMA, London.

British United Provident Association (1992) *A Guide to Private Consultant Practice.* BUPA, London.

British United Provident Association (1992) *Schedule of Procedures.* BUPA, London.

Calman K (1993) *Hospital Doctors: Training for the Future—Report of the Working Group on Specialist Medical Training.* Department of Health, London.

Income Data Services (1993) *Private Medical Insurance. Study no. 527.*

Laing W (1993) *Laing's Review of Private Healthcare.* Laing & Buisson, London.

Laing W (1992) *Healthcare Report: UK Private Specialists' Fees—Is the Price Right?* Norwich Union Healthcare, Norwich.

The Wyatt Company (1992) *Survey of Medical Benefits.* Wyatt, London.

6

Specialist Fees

Concern at the cost of specialist fees

Thirty years ago the public perception of private healthcare was centred on Harley Street. In those days the patient expected to pay a high price for the personal services of what he assumed to be a top specialist. The health insurers would most likely have reimbursed the costs involved, subject to overall benefit levels, without demur, having no clear idea at that time of what was the average cost of consultations and operations and whether the services of that specialist were expensive relative to those of his peers.

The situation has completely changed since that time. 70% of private treatment is now covered by health insurance. PMI is now a multi-million pound industry involving 12% of the population. The health insurers, being acutely aware of the running costs of their business, the ratio of income to expenditure, and the activities of their competitors, are determined to control costs, if not actually reduce them, and are focusing more and more attention on specialists' professional fees. Sophisticated computerized accounting systems provide the insurers with a wealth of data from which to extrapolate an average of fees charged for particular procedures and establish a yardstick against which the charges of individual specialists can be measured. In this way professional fees are being subjected to a degree of scrutiny never before contemplated. Although in theory the price of the specialist's services is the subject of a contract between the doctor and the patient with the consultant being free to charge what he likes, in practice it is the health insurers who have the greatest influence over what is charged.

Elements of professional fees

Before looking further at the context of this scrutiny and its effects, it may be useful to consider what specialists' professional fees are supposed to cover. The considerations involved may be summarized as follows:

Qualifications

Consideration of the specialist's qualifications is no longer an objective matter. As we have seen, there has been a heated debate recently among the medical establishment as to the relative value and significance of certain qualifications, most notably the EC Certificate of Specialist Training. In general, the most obvious criterion for excellence is the award of a fellowship such as the FRCP or FRCS. However, this is regarded by the insurers as less important than the holding of a substantive NHS consultant post.

Relevant experience

This is a more subjective factor. As we have seen there are many eminent private practitioners who, for various reasons, have not achieved some of the higher qualifications mentioned and yet are judged by their peers, and occasionally by the health insurers, to be of 'equivalent status' by virtue of their experience in a particular field.

The specialist's skill

This is wholly subjective. In the absence of proper audit there is nothing with which to gauge this other than by outcome and its concomitants: patient satisfaction and a good reputation among referring GPs. It remains to be seen whether more objective criteria can be devised via professional audit. The idea of professional league tables indicative of success rates among hospitals and individual surgeons is unlikely to be adopted in this country, as it has been in certain parts of the USA, but they should not be too readily dismissed (*see* Chapter 18).

Time expended/degree of difficulty

These are crucial considerations in setting fees for individual operations or procedures. They are subject to considerable variation. Some surgeons are meticulous about operations which others consider sufficiently routine to undertake a number of them in quick succession. Techniques also vary to a considerable degree. The operation to remove varicose veins, for example, is undertaken by both general surgeons and those specializing in vascular surgery, and views will often differ among them as to the degree of difficulty involved. It is known, for instance, that certain specialists can spend two hours on an operation on which some surgeons would spend 45 minutes. The surgeon taking the longer time might point to the cosmetically superior results of his work, but others would question whether this was necessary or justified the much higher price which he will consequently feel obliged to charge. As it happens, this is the one type of operation for which there is perhaps the greatest variation in fees charged. One health insurer calculated the range of variation to be about 60%, compared with a range of 10–20% for most other operations.

'Averaging out'

There is a feeling among many specialists, given expression in the BMA Guidelines, that the fee charged for a particular operation should be based on the usual or average cost of that operation when undertaken by that specialist. Some operations will be difficult and take longer than others. Although it is open to the specialist to charge a higher fee when an unexpectedly lengthy operation is involved, it is considered that the averaging out of most procedures is the fairest and easiest way to manage professional fees. This line of thinking would also involve including additional minor procedures which are a necessary preliminary to, or a routine consequence of, a particular major procedure being included within the standard fee, rather than listed separately.

Overheads

The cost of overheads should be built into the cost of any operation/ procedure. They include the cost of consulting rooms and utilities used, equipment/consumables, staff and assistants' salaries, and insurance including professional indemnity insurance.

Geographical location

In general it is recognized that the fees of provincial surgeons will be less than of those based in Central London. Provincial surgeons may well doubt whether the degree of differential is justified, but overheads are certainly higher in London, as are the costs of living. The health insurers have acknowledged the higher costs of treatment in London in the bandings for private hospitals. They are nevertheless questioning the justification for the differential insofar as it relates to the purported pre-eminence of London specialists over provincial colleagues. As a corollary to the averaging out of fees involved in operations, the BMA Guidelines have striven to postulate the average cost of an operation taking the country as a whole. They offer no distinction between London and elsewhere, taking the costs of both into account and averaging them out. Few specialists practising in London accept this approach.

Comparison with colleagues

Many practitioners setting up in private practice for the first time have no idea what to charge, and therefore base their fees on what their colleagues in the same specialty locally charge, however high or low these may happen to be in comparison with the average. Some specialists, especially those who undertake only a limited amount of private practice, often fail to increase their fees annually in line with inflation factors as might be expected. In contrast, others will increase their fees in accordance with inflation factors of their own devising, including many of the elements mentioned above, with religious punctuality.

The specialist's reputation

This is a curious phenomenon. Many interested in private practice have observed that patients often judge the work of a specialist by the level of his fees, assuming, without any justification, that those who charge most must by definition be the best. As one surgeon put it: 'The quickest way for me to go out of business would be to halve my fees.' This may be one reason why specialists in Harley Street continue to enjoy so much work among the non-insured population. Those for whom money is no object will find reassurance in the size of the fee charged by the doctor they consult, be he specialist or GP.

Amounts reimbursed by insurers

Despite all the aforesaid considerations it should be acknowledged that the amount of reimbursement by health insurers, principally BUPA, is one of the principal factors determining the level of fees charged. In his report *Private Specialist Fees—Is the Price Right?* independent healthcare consultant William Laing noted that the BUPA benefit levels are 'still the principal benchmark for the setting of specialists' fees'. It is believed the results of the MMC survey in 1993 will demonstrate this beyond peradventure.

The reasons for this are simple. By charging less or no more than the reimbursement levels prescribed in the BUPA schedule, the specialists concerned can expect to receive payment without difficulty. Charging higher fees, on the other hand, may be calculated to lead to disputes with BUPA and with other insurers, as well as with the patient concerned, over the shortfall between the fee due and the amount reimbursed. At the very least the practitioner may experience some delay in payment.

The assault on overcharging

There is a further dimension to the insurers' preoccupation with the cost of private specialist fees. This is the attempt to marginalize a few 'maverick' specialists who consistently charge way above the levels charged by the majority of their peers. The activities of this minority have caused the insurers many problems as a result of difficulties with patients arising from shortfalls between the fees charged by these specialists and benefits reimbursed. The medical directors or advisers to health insurance companies not infrequently write to such specialists querying the level of fees charged for particular procedures with reference to the BUPA or PPP schedules or the BMA Guidelines.

However, the insurers do not yet seem to have worked out the best way of dealing with those who refuse to be persuaded by such arguments. One idea mooted by BUPA was to compile an 'approved list' of specialists (not the same as the present list of approved specialists) for use by their corporate clients. This would be composed of only those whose fees were broadly in line with their benefit levels. An idea mooted by PPP, meanwhile, was to send letters to specialists whom they adjudged to be charging too much, and to advise their subscribers to enquire of the specialist if he has received any such letter before the consultation. Clearly both ideas are problematic.

While BUPA and PPP are clearly determined to isolate those charging way above average, they are anxious to do so without being seen to impede the patient's and his GP's freedom of choice. However, such moves are making it increasingly difficult to sustain the notion that such freedom of choice continues to exist, and gives the lie to the idea of a wholly indirect relationship between insurer and provider.

Effect of the BMA's guidelines

The assault on overcharging is not confined to the insurers. The BMA has likewise been concerned to eschew methods of charging which bring the profession and private practice into disrepute. The protagonists of the BMA Guidelines have made a concerted attempt to bring an end to the practice of charging separately for every minor procedure undertaken at a consultation. The Guidelines seek to discourage the practice of charging the same rate for each of several procedures undertaken sequentially during the same in-patient episode. They point out that the elements of overheads built into the price of a stand-alone procedure should not be repeated for each additional procedure. The wording of the introduction of the BMA Guidelines and its list of minor procedures which should attract only a 'modest fee in addition to the consultation rates', clearly attempt to put paid to such practices. As BUPA had done before them, the BMA later tried to produce a rough formula for dealing with operations, other than those normally undertaken bilaterally, which are undertaken at the same time as the first operation through the same 'portal of entry'.

Many of the smaller insurers use the BMA Guidelines when considering whether fees charged by specialists are 'reasonable', though they are clearly in no way as influential as the BUPA benefit levels. However, in his 1992 report for Norwich Union Healthcare, Laing noted the linkage of the BMA Guidelines to the level of increases in consultant remuneration awarded by the Doctors and Dentists Review Body, commenting that 'the BMA guidelines are therefore inflationary in tendency'. This perception may have contributed to the decision of the Office of Fair Trading to investigate the BMA Guidelines in 1992, an investigation which eventually resulted in its referral to the

Monopolies and Mergers Commission as part of a full-scale investigation of private consultant fees.

The Laing/Norwich Union report on specialist fees

The essential message of this report is that the price of specialist fees is too high. This conclusion was based on comparisons with other professions and fees charged by specialists in other developed countries using estimates of UK specialists' earnings derived from insurers' data. However, the fact that the results of the MMC's 1993 survey are believed to be at variance with these estimates may cast doubt on the validity of the report's conclusions.

The report begins by pointing to an alleged increase in the proportion of specialists' earnings derived from private practice from an estimated 13% in 1975 to 31% in 1990. This is based on an expenses figure of 15%, though allowing a higher figure of 25% gives only a smaller percentage share figure of 28% in 1990. A number of consultants queried those figures, pointing out that expenses could be as high as 50% (*see* Fig 6.1). The Hospital Consultants and Specialists Association later claimed that a survey of its members revealed an average of expenses in excess of 30% of fees received.

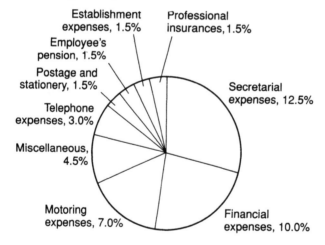

Total 43.0%

Figure 6.1: Purported example of specialist expenses. These figures are a purported breakdown of a consultant's earnings in the private sector. The remainder is taxed and profits must still pay for benefits such as a pension.

Taking his own estimate of consultants' gross private fee income at 1990 of £40 000 per annum, Laing deduced a projected mean net income of between £39 000 and £44 000, based on his own estimate of average expenses. Noting from BUPA's 1992 figures that 10% of private consultants earn 46% of the benefits paid out he calculated the net private practice income for the top 10% to be in the order of £93 000 to £105 000 per annum.

However, initial reports suggest that the 1993 MMC survey found the median gross earnings of NHS consultants from private practice to be much lower, at about £25 000 per annum, producing a net income of approximately £18 000. It is believed the highest decile were found to be earning around £91 000 per annum gross (£67 000 net).

According to Laing, the earnings of NHS consultants practising part-time in private medicine would be less than those of senior barristers, though substantially more than senior architects and junior legal counsel. If the findings of the MMC survey referred to above are confirmed, these broad comparisons may require revision.

Reputed earnings of 'whole-time equivalents'

For the purposes of comparison with other countries, it is the earnings of those in full-time private practice or 'whole-time equivalents' (WTEs) to which the Laing report accords the greatest significance, though the report calculates the number of specialists practising solely in private practice to be less than 1000 (the BMA believes it may be as few as 500) compared with the total of 12 000 plus NHS specialists undertaking private practice. The estimated net earnings of WTEs are based on a survey of surgical activities in independent hospitals. However, this takes no account of physicians' and anaesthetists' fees, which are admittedly lower, so that if half of those individual private consultants are surgeons, one could be talking of as few as 250–500 individuals at most. These, according to Laing's estimates, could be earning approximately £3000 a day as at 1990, on approximately 110 operating days a year, giving £330 000 a year, plus £70 000 in consultation fees, making a potential gross earnings total of £400 000 per annum and net earnings of between £300 000 to £340 000 per annum, after deducting expenses of between 15 and 25%.

It is generally accepted by all commentators that there may be a few specialists, perhaps no more than a dozen, who are able to earn more than £400 000 per annum. On the other hand several thousand specialists may be earning less than £1000 per year, because of the limited amount of private practice available in their specialty or particular locality.

It is on the basis of his estimate of WTE earnings, and on a comparison of fees charged for a selection of common operations that, having noted the difficulty of comparing 'like with like', Laing concluded that UK surgeons' fees are 60% higher than US Medicare fees, Spanish private medical insurance fees and those recommended by the Australian Medical Association; four times higher than German and Canadian Medicare fees, and 170% more than French private practice rates.

Is the price too high?

Laing concluded his report by saying that specialist private practice fees 'are probably considerably higher than necessary to ensure an adequate supply of top level specialists skills for the insured population'. Many specialists found the figures on which this conclusion was based unconvincing, and it may be that the findings of the MMC survey justify their scepticism. However, whatever the size of the disparity between the real cost of private specialist fees in the UK and other developed nations, Laing undoubtedly had a valid point when he noted that these differences may be viewed as a 'subsidy' which UK medical insurers are indirectly paying to the NHS, the effect of which is to maintain surgeons' overall income at a level comparable with those of surgeons overseas.

We have already observed that the universality of NHS provision has determined that private healthcare is a high price luxury commodity or corporate perk for a minority of the population. The question 'why are private fees so much higher than the equivalent proportion of those consultants' NHS salaries?' might be countered with a further question: 'Is there any reason why doctors devoting substantially the whole of their professional time to the NHS should not seek to maximize income from the limited time available to them to undertake private practice?' Moreover, given that the NHS is their priority, why should consultants seek to charge less to those who are not prepared to take their chances in waiting for NHS treatment like the 88% of the population who have no alternative?

Market imperfections and the 'level playing field'

In mid-1993 the stock of economic commentary on this subject was further enhanced by the publication of a report, again sponsored by Norwich Union Healthcare, by the National Economic Research Associates (NERA). Central to this report was research into the effect on specialist fees of the BMA's guidelines which, at face value, appeared to validate the insurers' concerns by demonstrating how fee-setting by some individual specialists tended to be clustered around the BMA's postulated averages, rather than being spaced out as one might expect in a genuinely unregulated market. However, the report notes that 'There are certain basic imperfections in the market' and that 'the BMA schedules are only one of several practices which affect competition between providers in the market for private medical services'.

What the report also manages to demonstrate beyond doubt is the complexity of the way in which this market (or, as it later describes it, the multiplicity of separate markets) manages to function, and how difficult it is to control, given the absence of a level playing field between public and private sector treatment. Both the Laing report and NERA also demonstrate that the market in private specialists' services is, by its nature, a nature determined by its relationship with the NHS, an imperfect market. There is therefore little the health insurers or anyone else can do, given the prevailing system, to make this market function in accordance with classic theories of market economics: hence the desire to find ways of radically altering the present system (*see* Chapter 18).

The MMC Inquiry

The MMC began its investigation into private medical services in September 1992, announcing shortly after that it was to concentrate its attention on specialist services only. As part of the enquiry, the MMC undertook a postal survey of some 4600 consultants chosen at random from across a broad range of specialties, and sought to interview a randomly chosen sample of 470 specialists about the means by which their fees were determined, the considerations involved and the amounts they derived from private practice as compared with their NHS remuneration. The full results of this survey, the largest of its kind ever undertaken in the field of private specialist practice, were unknown at the time this book went to press.

However, in a letter to consultants on completion of their survey in the summer of 1993, the Commission indicated that it had determined 'that some NHS consultants are part of and benefit from what the Fair Trading Act 1973 defines as a "complex monopoly situation".' The basis for this finding was that some 9500 or so NHS consultants were believed in 1992 to have fixed more than 50% of their fees for private medical services at or very close to either the BMA Guidelines or the BUPA or PPP Schedules of Reimbursement.

Accordingly the MMC was to consider whether the continued publication of such schedules was in the public interest, with a view to making recommendations to the Secretary of State for Trade and Industry regarding any remedial action it deemed to be appropriate.

It must be assumed that the relative degree of adherence to the respective fee schedules will be all-important; and if initial reports, which suggest that the MMC survey confirmed a tendency for charges to converge on the BUPA maxima rather than the scales contained in the BMA's guidelines, are correct, it may leave the Commission in something of a quandary. It is taken for granted by competition authorities like the MMC that publication by a professional organization of advice to its members about fees they may charge is anti-competitive and 'in restraint of trade'. Other professions (eg architects and surveyors), which had sought to regulate prices for services charged by their members, had already been taken to task by the OFT and MMC.

However, while it may be considered by many to be perverse, it is a fact that the concept of 'monopsony', the attempt by purchasers acting in concert to control prices, is not one which competition authorities necessarily find reprehensible. They argue that the use of monopolistic powers by purchasers, even if unfair, will generally be found to be in the public interest in that the result will be lower prices which benefit the consumer.

Having established that a 'complex monopoly' exists, therefore, it will be interesting to note where the weight of the Commission's criticism will fall. Will the MMC be forced to absolve BUPA and PPP and castigate only the BMA by ruling that it suspend publication of its guidelines? The MMC's conclusions will hinge on what it adjudges to be in the public interest, and the Commission will have to ponder whether suppression of information about fees is in the public interest or whether the public would be better served by dissemination of accurate and independently assessed data on what fees are actually charged by private specialists.

References and further reading

Blair P and National Economic Research Associates (1993) *Healthcare Report: Reforming the Private Sector*. Norwich Union Healthcare, Norwich.

British Medical Association (1992) *Private Consultant Work: BMA Guidelines 1992*. BMA, London.

British United Provident Association (1992) *A Guide to Private Consultant Practice*. BUPA, London.

British United Provident Association (1992) *Schedule of Procedures*. BUPA, London.

Calman K (1993) *Hospital Doctors: Training for the Future—Report of the Working Group on Specialist Medical Training*. Department of Health, London.

Income Data Services (1993) *Private Medical Insurance. Study no. 527*.

Laing W (1992) *Healthcare Report: UK Private Specialists' Fees—Is the Price Right?* Norwich Union Healthcare, Norwich.

Laing W (1993) *Laing's Review of Private Healthcare*. Laing & Buisson, London.

The Wyatt Company (1992) *Survey of Medical Benefits*. Wyatt, London.

7

Legal Considerations

GMC registration

Having considered the historical, professional and economic contexts in which private medical practice is undertaken, we now need to look at the legal context, to understand what legal requirements have to be complied with in order to practise medicine privately in the UK.

To begin with it should be understood that one must be fully registered with the General Medical Council (GMC) in accordance with the provisions of the Medical Act 1983. Doctors with provisional or limited registration cannot practise in their own right without supervision. Doctors who are citizens of EC countries are entitled by virtue of section 3 (10) of the Act to be fully registered if they hold one or more recognized primary qualifications obtained in a member state of the EC. Other overseas doctors can be fully registered if they satisfy the GMC that they have the necessary qualifications and experience defined in sections 19 and 20 of the Act.

Having registered, a doctor is free to offer his services to patients, to advertise those services, subject to GMC guidelines, and to treat and prescribe for patients, to refer them to hospital, and charge patients or third parties for medical services.

Under UK law it is not an offence for a non-medically qualified person to provide medical assistance or treatment to another person with the latter's consent. However, it is an offence to purport to be a medically qualified and registered doctor if not so qualified and registered.

Prescribing medicinal products

The ability to prescribe medication is a prerequisite of medical practice. The rules which govern the private practitioner in this regard are exactly the same as those by which NHS doctors are obliged to abide. The basic rules are set out as follows.

Section 58(2)(a) of the Medicines Act 1968 provides that certain medicinal products may only be sold in accordance with 'a prescription given by an appropriate practitioner'. The 'appropriate practitioner' in this context means a doctor who is a registered medical practitioner. The question of what products are covered by the Act and what must be contained in the prescription are dealt with in the Medicines (Products Other Than Veterinary Drugs) (Prescriptions Only) Order 1983 as amended by the Medicines (Products Other Than Veterinary Drugs) (General Sales List) Order 1984. The list of medicinal products controlled in this way is contained in the Schedule to the Regulations which is amended from time to time. Under the Medicines Act any prescription issued must be written in ink or be otherwise indelible and be signed in ink by the practitioner with his own name. It should also include the following particulars:

- the address of the practitioner
- the date
- the category of practitioner (eg registered medical practitioner)
- the name, address and age (if under 12) of the patient

The prescription cannot be dispensed if it is more than six months old unless it is a repeat prescription, in which case the first dispensing is not to take place more than six months after the date of the prescription. If a repeatable prescription does not specify how many times it is to be dispensed there can be only two dispensings of it, except in the case of oral contraceptives which may be dispensed up to six times before the six months are up. In an emergency, prescription-only drugs which are not 'controlled', may be dispensed without a prescription if a doctor requests the same and undertakes the supply of a prescription within 72 hours.

Controlled drugs

The Misuse of Drugs Regulations 1985 define the classes of person who are authorized to supply and possess controlled drugs as specified in the Misuse of Drugs Act 1971 while acting in their professional capacities, and lays down the conditions under which these activities may be carried out. The Regulations divide drugs into five schedules, each specifying the requirements governing such activities as import, export, production, supply, possession, prescribing and record-keeping which apply to them.

Regulation 19 of the Misuse of Drugs Regulations requires any person authorized to possess or supply a controlled drug to maintain a register and an approved form of a quantity of all controlled drugs obtained and supplied, including any administered personally. A separate part of the register is to be maintained for each class of drugs mentioned in the schedules. Regulation 20 specifies the requirements for maintaining the register. All controlled drugs must be kept in a locked receptacle which can only be opened by the doctor or with his authority. In addition to the usual details required, a prescription for a controlled drug must specify the strength of the preparation, the dose to be taken and the quantity of the preparation in both words and figures.

Supply of medicinal products by doctors

Section 9 of the Medicines Act 1968 provides some exemption from the general prohibition on commercial supply or sale of medicinal products without a product licence for doctors, dentists and veterinary surgeons. Section 9 states that the restrictions in section 7 do not apply to anything done by a doctor which:

> *'a) Relates to a medicinal product specifically prepared, or especially imported by him or to his order, for administration to a particular patient of his, and consists of manufacturing or assembling, or procuring the manufacture or assembly of, the product, or selling or supplying, or procuring the sale or supply of, the product to that patient or to a person under whose care that patient is, or*
> *b) When the doctor does likewise at the request of another doctor or dentist for administration to a patient of their own.'*

Dispensing of medicinal products by a doctor

The Medicines Act 1968 empowers all doctors to dispense medication, provided that there is compliance with the terms of the Act with regard to such issues as safe custody of medicines, record-keeping, labelling and standards of containers. Doctors providing pharmaceutical services to patients are required to provide them in appropriate containers. In accordance with the Medicines (Child Safety) Regulations 1975–76, all containers used for the supply of medication should be reclosable and child-resistant, unless the patient is elderly or disabled and would have difficulty in opening a child-resistant container. A 5 ml plastic measuring spoon shall be supplied with every oral liquid medicine unless the patient already has a spoon or the manufacturer's pack contains one.

The Medicines (Labelling) Regulations 1976–1985 further require that any medication dispensed, whether by a doctor or on the instructions of a doctor, must be appropriately labelled. Such a label must include:

- the name of the person to whom the medicine is to be given
- the name and address of the supplier (the doctor, if he has dispensed)
- the date the prescription was dispensed
- the words 'keep out of reach of children'.

There is no legal requirement, but it is deemed to be good practice, to include the name of the preparation, instructions for use and any other appropriate warnings.

Product liability

Part 1 of the Consumer Protection Act 1987 removes the need for a person who suffers damage as a result of taking a drug to prove negligence. It is now only necessary to prove that the product was defective and that any damage caused was the result of such a defect. The liability falls on the manufacturer or importer. Where neither of these is identifiable, however, liability will rest with the supplier unless he can identify a person higher up the distribution chain, eg the wholesaler. It is therefore imperative that doctors maintain a record of each drug supplied to every patient. This should be kept in the patient's record. Records should also be kept of all invoices so as to identify the source of every drug. These records should be kept for at least 11 years.

Doctor v patient

Having looked at the legal background to some of the services provided to private patients, it may now be helpful to consider the nature of the relationship between the private doctor and his patient in legal terms.

It is axiomatic that a private patient enters into a contract with a doctor for treatment. Patient and doctor are free to negotiate the terms of such a contract. It is rare for a written contract to exist between doctor and patient; rather, the terms will be implicit in their relationship. If the doctor fulfils his part of the contract but the patient does not, ie by not paying for his treatment, the doctor may have recourse to the law to sue for recovery in a small claims court (*see* Chapter 13). If the doctor does not fulfil his part of the contract, various judicial remedies can be considered.

Many patients assume that there must be some medical regulatory body whom they can approach if they have a specific complaint about a private practitioner. The simple fact is that the only body with any ability to discipline a private practitioner is the GMC, and then only in a case of serious professional misconduct (*see* Chapter 8). The GMC has for some time been

considering proposals for a system of dealing with complaints about professional competence involving a form of performance review, but its proposals
are some way from being finalized. Patients are occasionally appalled to dis-
cover that there is no organization to whom they can complain if they consider their private doctor's bill to be excessive. The fact is there is no
mechanism by which bills can be so investigated. It is always a case of 'caveat
emptor'.

Patient v doctor

There are two grounds on which to seek legal redress against private medical
practitioners: *battery* (ie assault) or *negligence*.

With battery the issue of consent is all important. The patient only has to
establish that the doctor touched him without consent. He does not have to
show that any loss or damage resulted from an unlawful act. Damages can be
awarded for all direct consequences of the battery.

Negligence is a complex issue. It is defined in law as the breach of a duty to
use reasonable care as a result of which there is damage to another. To succeed in proving negligence in order to sue for damages the aggrieved patient
will have to establish, on the balance of probabilities: (1) that a legal duty of
care was owed by the doctor to the patient; (2) that the doctor was in breach
of that duty, ie his behaviour fell short of the standard required by law, *and* it
was reasonably foreseeable that the negligent behaviour in question could
damage the plaintiff; and (3) that there is a causal link between the behaviour
and damage which must be proved to have been sustained as a result.

However serious a negligent act may be, it is a matter for the criminal law
only if the victim dies. Gross negligence or recklessness causing death can
amount to manslaughter. The burden of proof required to establish criminal
liability is more than that required for civil liability. The doctor must have
shown such disregard for the life and safety of others as to amount to a crime
against the State and conduct deserving of punishment.

Risk management

In the USA, where lawsuits based on medical negligence are commonplace,
medical practitioners have developed a concept known as risk management
which aims to reduce the risk of therapeutic mishaps or adverse outcomes and
thereby reduce the risk of legal proceedings. The basis of this concept is what
is referred to as the 'four Cs': communication, consent and counselling, competence and case notes. The last two need no particular explanation. The

recommended approach to communication and consent can best be summarized as follows:

- providing personal protocols for preoperative and postoperative management of patients and familiarity with hospital protocols

- giving clear and concise instructions to the nursing staff and staff in operating theatres used

- communicating regularly and courteously with patients and relatives

- providing the fullest information about proposed treatment and operations, eg by information sheets

- giving proper warnings of the possibility of significant complications or risks

- discussing alternative methods of therapy with the patient or relatives

- ensuring the patient has time to properly consider what is involved and offer informed consent

- obtaining of signed consent forms as a permanent record and acknowledgment that proper counselling has taken place

- explaining readily whenever part of the treatment does not go according to plan.

Medico-legal experts suggest that, if followed, this regimen will considerably reduce the risk of a malpractice suit being successful. There is another piece of advice which is the corollary to the regimen of risk management: if a mistake is made or something goes wrong for which the practitioner is directly or indirectly responsible, he must not only be prepared to explain what has happened to the patient and relatives, but also to offer an apology. It has been proved on many occasions that a swift and sympathetic response and an admission of regret are sometimes all that are needed to avoid a potentially damaging and costly legal dispute.

Professional indemnity

In view of all that we have revealed about the legal pitfalls and perpetual risks of litigation facing the independent medical practitioner, it should come as no surprise that one of the most important preliminaries to setting up in private practice is to obtain the appropriate professional indemnity insurance or 'medical defence' cover. It is perhaps curious that practising doctors are not required by law to have professional indemnity insurance. However, it would be a rash individual indeed who attempted to practise without it. The UK is spared the complete obsession with medical negligence evidenced in the USA, but accusations of medical negligence are nevertheless a common phenomenon and every doctor must be prepared to face the prospect of litigation at least once in his career. We have already seen that proof of adequate indemnity insurance is a prerequisite for the granting of admitting rights to private hospitals. Accordingly, it is strongly recommended by all representative bodies that doctors obtain sufficient defence cover.

Until comparatively recently, all practising doctors had to take out professional indemnity insurance regarding every aspect of their professional activity, though the Department of Health reimbursed most of the costs incurred in this respect by their employed staff. Then in 1990, following lengthy negotiations with representatives of the profession and the medical defence organizations, the Department of Health agreed to assume total responsibility for acts of negligence committed by their hospital and community health employees (including consultants). Funds were established for this purpose, supplemented by monies which the defence societies agreed to make over to the Department as they relinquished responsibility for the activities of their hospital and community health subscribers.

However, the responsibility of the Department of Health only extended to acts committed in the course of NHS employment. It was therefore accepted that doctors would need to continue to maintain defence cover in respect of private practice and for 'good Samaritan' acts. The introduction of NHS indemnity did not, therefore, bring about the demise of the medical defence organizations: rather it brought about a rationalization of their activities. They have not abandoned their expertise in dealing with NHS hospital practice, since they now act as advisers to health authorities; not surprisingly, however, they have been able to concentrate more resources on private practice.

GPs were of course excluded from the new arrangements, since they were independent contractors rather than salaried employees. The cost of their defence cover was, in any case, quite small relative to the high-risk occupation of hospital medicine. While GPs currently have professional indemnity for their NHS activities, taking on private patients will not affect the nature or cost of the cover they need. For hospital practitioners, medical defence cover for private practice may prove to be a not inconsiderable expense (although it can be claimed against tax). The amounts payable will vary depending on the nature and amount of activity. Defence cover for the surgical specialties will obviously be higher and this is something to be taken into account in the setting of professional fees.

There are three medical defence organizations: the Medical Defence Union, the Medical Protection Society and the Medical and Dental Defence Union of Scotland (the latter has only recently thrown its doors open to non-Scottish graduates). Their addresses appear in the Appendix. While some insurance companies have attempted to offer cheap indemnity insurance to GPs, there are no serious alternatives to these three organizations. Their knowledge of medico-legal issues is unrivalled, except perhaps by the BMA, which of course represents the profession's interests in every field and, indeed, works co-operatively with the defence organizations in individual cases.

References and further reading

British Medical Association (1993) *Health Authority Indemnity* (Guidance note).

General Medical Council (1992) *Professional Conduct and Discipline: Fitness to Practice*. GMC, London.

Medical Ethics Committee, BMA (1992) *Rights and Responsibilities of Doctors*. BMA, London.

8

Ethical Considerations

The disciplinary role of the GMC

We have already mentioned that the General Medical Council is the body with statutory responsibility for the regulation and discipline of the medical profession. This responsibility is derived from the Medical Acts (the latest of which is the Medical Act 1983). In accordance with its provisions all doctors are bound to abide by the rules which the GMC prescribes from time to time for the conduct of the profession, on pain of disciplinary action. The GMC's rules are described in a booklet entitled *Professional Conduct and Discipline: Fitness to Practice*, known colloquially as the 'Blue Book'.

Whereas NHS doctors are bound by the rules appertaining to their contracts and terms of service, as well as by the rules of the GMC, doctors acting in a private capacity need only have regard to the latter, except when undertaking private practice in an NHS hospital. The GMC has the power to prevent a doctor from continuing to practise medicine either by suspending or by erasing his name from the medical register. Suspension is, by definition, temporary, being seen as a corrective measure necessary to ensure compliance during a period not exceeding three years with whatever requirements the GMC's Professional Conduct Committee sees fit to impose for the protection of the public or in the doctor's own interest. Erasure remains effective unless and until the doctor makes a successful application for restoration to the register.

There are two grounds on which the Professional Conduct Committee can suspend or strike off a doctor's name: conviction of a criminal offence or proof of 'serious professional misconduct'. The Committee is bound to accept criminal conviction as proof that the doctor was guilty of the offence of which he was charged. In matters involving allegations of serious professional misconduct the circumstances must be looked into by a Preliminary Screening Committee which has the power either to dismiss the case, postpone consideration pending amelioration of the situation or, where the Committee believe the allegation is substantiated, refer the matter to the Professional Conduct Committee to decide.

The Professional Conduct Committee will invite submissions from the accused doctor, including character references, testimonials and details of mitigating circumstances as well as a submission from the parties making the allegation. It will then consider the evidence and oral submissions from the parties at a public hearing. Parties may be represented at the hearing by lawyers and call witnesses as in any other kind of judicial hearing. An appeal against a direction from the Committee that the doctor's name be erased or suspended from the register can only be made on a point of law on direct application within 28 days of the decision to the Judicial Committee of the Privy Council.

Serious professional misconduct

The question of what is involved in serious professional misconduct has been the subject of much discussion recently both within the GMC and outside it. The categories of behaviour which are felt to justify this description are as follows:

- neglect or disregard by doctors of their professional responsibilities to patients for their care and treatment
- abuse of professional privileges or skills
- improper behaviour: ie conduct 'derogatory to the reputation of the medical profession'
- improper comment on professional colleagues
- improper advertising of doctors' services.

Let us consider these categories in more detail.

Standards of care

Standards of care may be easy to define in the abstract, but in practice they exercise the judgemental abilities of the Professional Conduct Committee of the GMC in individual cases to a considerable extent. Generally speaking the GMC is not concerned with errors of diagnosis or treatment, or matters which give rise to allegations of negligence in the civil courts, except where the doctor's conduct in a particular case involves a blatant disregard or neglect of professional responsibility.

Abuse of professional privileges

Such abuse in this context includes inappropriate prescription of controlled drugs or inappropriate issue of medical certificates (eg for fraudulent purposes); improper disclosure of confidential information about patients; exerting pressure on patients to lend the doctor money or perform favours; and having a sexual relationship with a patient.

Conduct derogatory to the profession

This may involve personal misuse of alcohol or other drugs or indecent or violent behaviour. It may also include dishonesty and financial impropriety. Examples of this cited in the 'Blue Book' include charging of patient's fees for in-patient or out-patient treatment when they may not properly be regarded as private patients, and 'other improper arrangements calculated to extend or otherwise benefit' the doctor, such as 'pressure by a specialist to persuade a patient to accept private treatment by reliance upon representations about the comparative availability of treatment under the NHS and privately'.

One of the areas which the GMC views with considerable concern in this context is the notion of 'fee-splitting'. An example of this might be if a specialist were to agree to give part of his professional fee for treating a patient to the GP who referred that patient to him. Both doctors in this situation would be liable for disciplinary action. However, it would also be regarded as a potentially disciplinary matter for a GP to accept remuneration from any party who stood to benefit financially from the referral of one of his patients, whether NHS or private. The importance of declaring to the patient any financial interest which a doctor may have in an institution to which he intends to refer the patient has already been noted but is worth emphasizing here. Doctors must at all times endeavour to act, and be seen to be acting, in the best interests of the patient.

Improper comments about colleagues

This is bound up with advertising, which is a major subject dealt with in detail below.

Advertising

For many years the GMC declared virtually any advertising of medical services to be unbecoming of the dignity of the profession. Following pressure from the Monopolies and Mergers Commission the GMC was forced to abandon this rather anachronistic stance, and it issued new guidelines in 1990. Their reluctance is aptly summarized in the following extract from *Professional Conduct and Discipline: Fitness to Practice*:

> 'The promotion of doctors' medical services as if the provision of
> medical care were no more than a commercial activity is likely

both to undermine public trust in the medical profession and, over time, to diminish the standards of medical care which patients have a right to expect.'

The new GMC guidelines are much more permissive for GPs than for specialists. They make a distinction between, on the one hand, making available factual information about doctors' qualifications and services, and, on the other, promotional material which, while extolling the virtues of individual practitioners, may by implication denigrate other doctors or hold them up to unfair comparisons. In general it is expected that advertising by doctors should be consistent with the requirements of the British Code of Advertising Practice in being 'legal, decent, honest and truthful'. Information provided by a doctor about his practice should also be accurate and not capable of being misinterpreted. It should not compare or contrast the quality of services with that provided by other doctors, nor imply that those advertised can achieve results from treatment not achievable by others. Doctors have a duty to ensure throughout that any advertising with which they are associated does not put patients at risk or mislead them in any way.

Advertising by GPs

Lists containing factual information about NHS GPs are now routinely available in public places like libraries. These can include details of private services. As the lists are often provided by Family Health Services Authorities, private GPs may have difficulty in ensuring that details of their practices are made available in this way. They are at liberty, however, to provide the public with practice leaflets giving factual information about themselves, their services and practice arrangements, including, if they wish, a statement about their approach to medical practice. These may be distributed on an unsolicited basis within the area in which they practice, provided this does not put the recipients under any kind of pressure.

GPs may publish factual information about their services in the press, directories or other media but services should not be advertised by means of unsolicited visits or telephone calls either by the doctors themselves or others acting on their behalf with the specific aim of recruiting patients. Such activities may render the doctor liable to GMC disciplinary proceedings.

When advertising in local or national directories like Yellow Pages, entries should be in normal bold typeface or 'boxed', but when advertising in the press, GPs are advised to be wary of allowing their services to be presented in a promotional or laudatory manner. They may be held to account for the overall effect of such features if they imply disparagement of other doctors or their facilities. TV and radio advertising of medical services, though theoretically possible, is virtually unknown, and may pose even greater risks of being regarded as promotional or misleading.

Practice leaflets

A GP practice leaflet may contain the usual personal and professional details, ie name, sex, medical qualifications and date of first registration as a doctor. It may also include practice information such as:

- consultation times
- whether there is an appointment system and, if so, the method of obtaining urgent and non-urgent appointments and domiciliary visits
- how services are provided when the doctor is not available (through deputies etc)
- arrangements for obtaining repeat prescriptions (and dispensing, if a dispensing practice)
- details of other staff assisting and their roles
- details of the normal practice area
- additional services provided by the doctor, eg maternity, contraception or minor surgery services, together with details of special clinics (frequency, duration and purpose).

GP leaflets may include commercial advertising to reduce production costs. The BMA suggests that this should not relate to other health care activities like pharmacists, nursing homes, private hospitals or clinics since this may imply that those institutions have the endorsement of the doctor in question. Nor should it relate to businesses in which the doctor or a near relative has a financial interest.

Advertising by specialists

Since being taken to task by the MMC in its report on advertising in 1989, the GMC has had no objection to information about specialist services being provided to GPs and other professional colleagues. However it prohibits providing such information directly to the public except in very limited circumstances. The GMC explains the decision to allow dissemination of factual information to GPs as being necessary to facilitate the referral system. The prohibition on advertising to the public is intended to protect individual patients who are sufficiently ill to need consultant advice and who may there-fore be more susceptible to external pressures.

The information that specialists are permitted to provide to colleagues should be confined to factual details of services provided and practice ar-rangements. Such material should not claim superiority for the specialist's personal qualifications, experience or skill. These principles apply equally to specialists working in the NHS and in private practice. The name, profes-sional qualifications, address and telephone number of the specialist may be included in national and local directories but not otherwise made available to the general public. As regards entries in telephone directories, heavy type is not considered acceptable.

The restrictions on advertising even apply to the door-plate displayed out-side a consultant's rooms. Such a plate would be acceptable if modest in size and form, showing no more than the doctor's name and qualifications. It would be unacceptable ethically to put any descriptive wording on the plate, except the consultant's specialty if this is not readily apparent from his quali-fications. Anything which suggests that the consultant has unique personal abilities which are likely to attract patients, or seeks to promote professional advantage or financial benefit, will be construed as promotional and contrary to GMC rules.

Communication with GPs

It is quite proper for a specialist setting up in private practice for the first time to let GPs in his area know if his existence and availability. He may best do this by preparing a simple standard letter, eg:

> 'Mr R G Jones-Smyth, FRCS, presents his compliments and wishes to inform you that he is available for private consultation at [address of consulting room and telephone number] or at [home address and telephone number]. Requests for appoint-ments should be made by telephoning his secretary on [telephone number].'

Where the specialty is not apparent from the degree or diplomas it can also be defined. For example an FRCP may wish to indicate that he is a rheumatol-ogist or dermatologist etc. It would also be permissible for a psychiatrist with a special interest in psychotherapy, for instance, to indicate this interest. Some doctors may regard the expression 'presents his compliments' as ab-struse and antiquarian. Any polite modern form of address may be used as an alternative.

Communication with health insurers

For the reasons detailed in Chapter 5, it is essential for the newly appointed consultant setting up in private practice to write to the principal health insurers (whose addresses are given in the Appendix) indicating that he has the necessary credentials to meet their criteria for specialist recognition. He may thereby obtain confirmation from them of acceptance as 'an approved specialist'. This will prevent arguments from occurring later. As we have already seen, a specialist who is not able to meet those criteria can expect to experience a great deal of difficulty with insured patients, and should always check the status of such patients before commencing treatment so that they are left in no doubt as to his situation.

Advertising by groups of doctors and independent organizations

Associations of doctors are now allowed to release lists of their members on request to members of the public, provided they make it clear that those listed are not the only doctors qualified to practise in that specialty or branch of medicine, and that inclusion in the list does not imply any recommendation by that association.

Some private hospitals, screening centres, private clinics, nursing homes or advisory centres may also advertise medical services to the general public. Their ability to do so is governed by the same rules applying to GP services. Advertisements should not make adverse comparisons with the NHS or other organizations. They should not claim superiority for the professional services offered by doctors within such organizations. It should also be understood that the GMC considers it inappropriate for certain services (eg abortion) offered by private organizations to be advertised directly to the general public.

A doctor who has a professional or financial relationship with such an organization, or who simply uses its facilities, will bear a measure of responsibility for its advertising. Ignorance of the content of such advertising is no defence, should the advertising fail to conform to the standards set by the GMC. Such doctors are advised to satisfy themselves that any advertising does conform to these guidelines.

Some ethical concerns: GPs

Intraprofessional relationships

In Chapter 2 we noted that a small number of patients may choose to have both an NHS and a private GP. This can lead to problems where the patient who has consulted the GP privately asks the NHS GP to prescribe drugs in relation to the condition treated privately. The GMC and the BMA both make it clear in their ethical guidance that it is preferable for one doctor, ideally a GP, to be fully informed about and to be responsible for overall management of a patient's treatment. In cases where responsibility is shared, liaison between health professionals is desirable and the effective management of the patient's condition should be the foremost consideration of each doctor.

However, the fact remains that many NHS GPs may well refuse to prescribe in the circumstances described above, on the grounds that the private practitioner had assumed responsibility for management of the patient's condition and that the patient, having decided to go private, should accept the consequences of that decision and agree to pay privately for medication prescribed by that practitioner.

Private minor surgery

When Norwich Union Healthcare proposed to allow GPs to charge for private minor surgery, it was pointed out that GPs' terms of service forbade them to charge their own patients for or receive remuneration in respect of such treatment. It was therefore proposed that GPs refer appropriate patients to other GPs. This raised the possibility of reciprocal referrals, a concept which runs perilously close to the collusion deprecated by the GMC in its 'Blue book'. In recognition of the potential ethical difficulty, the BMA drew up a statement of guidance on the provision of private minor surgery services.

Charges for referral

We have already noted the resentment of GPs at being unable to charge for private referrals of their NHS patients (*see* Chapter 2). Health insurers are, in the main, conversant with the ethical and contractual constraints on GPs and any GP seeking remuneration from either an insured patient or direct from an insurer runs the risk of being reported to the GMC.

Some ethical concerns: specialists

Soliciting for private work

We have already noted that it is regarded as 'conduct derogatory to the profession' for a specialist to persuade a patient to accept private treatment by reliance upon representations about the comparative availability of treatment under the NHS and privately. It is also unethical for a specialist to seek, during the course of an NHS consultation, to arrange to treat a patient privately. This must be arranged separately from the NHS consultation to avoid any accusations that the specialist is seeking to extend his private practice by improper means.

Validation of 'six-week' insurance schemes

An ethical dilemma frequently adduced by specialists concerns validation of claims for treatment costs which may not be strictly allowable under the terms of the health insurance schemes in question. This has been a particular concern with regards to the operation of the so-called 'six-week' schemes, such as that operated by PPP in conjunction with the Automobile Association and BUPA's 'Healthchoice' scheme. What these schemes have in common is that the patient can only obtain reimbursement for private treatment of conditions for which there is a waiting-list of more than six weeks for treatment on the NHS.

It often transpires that patients assure specialists that treatment is covered by health insurance and only come to them after the event with claim forms requiring the specialist's signature indicating that the waiting-list for treatment was more than six weeks, when in fact this may not be the case. The specialist is then faced with the dilemma of either refusing to sign, and risk incurring the wrath of the patient, or putting his signature to a fraudulent claim. The BMA has complained to the providents about the invidious position which this type of scheme puts specialists in. The companies concerned have offered reassurance and guidance in the literature relevant to the scheme. However the only real solution is for the practitioner to enquire more closely of the patient before the event as to the scheme under which he is seeking treatment.

What these schemes also fail to address is the fact that, in many instances, hospitals can only speculate about the duration of the waiting-list in question. However, as NHS hospitals are encouraged to reduce waiting-lists it is clear that the ultimate benefactors will be the insurers, for whom the necessity to pay out benefits will be reduced accordingly.

Charging for insured and non-insured patients

A more general ethical concern, and one which is not easy to resolve, is the question of whether specialists should charge non-insured patients less than insured patients. A number of specialists routinely adjust their fees according to what they understand to be their patients' financial circumstances. The health insurers do not look sympathetically at this approach, and their concerns may be shared by the MMC. However, many in the profession would vigorously defend their rights to waive their fees where circumstances merit it, though it is less easy to justify inflated costs sometimes charged to foreign nationals who have come to the UK seeking treatment. In the absence of any organization responsible for regulating private fees, there is little which can be done about this.

Charging medical colleagues

It is of course an old tradition that doctors will not charge colleagues or their dependants for treatment. This was once included in the BMA's handbook of medical ethics, but it is now recognized as being a matter of etiquette rather than ethics, and there are many specialists today who refuse to waive fees for what may be long and difficult operations performed on doctors with whom they may have had no prior personal acquaintance. The BMA recently sought to encourage doctors to abide by this tradition, noting that the health insurance schemes operating for its members depend to a large extent on savings arising from it (*see* Chapter 15).

Debt recovery

Finally there is a perennial debate about the ethics of debt recovery (*see* Chapter 13). A minority of doctors still believe that pursuance of debts for treatment is demeaning and unworthy of their attention, and those who are members or fellows of the Royal College of Physicians are forbidden to take legal action for this purpose. However, the majority recognize that it is a fact that patients are no less likely to default on payment of debts than any other group of individuals, and that private doctors as small businessmen must respond accordingly.

References and further reading

General Medical Council (1990) *Guidance for Doctors on Advertising*. (Guidance note).

General Medical Council (1992) *Professional Conduct and Discipline: Fitness to Practice*. GMC, London.

Medical Ethics Committee, BMA (1991) *Guidelines to Doctors on Advertising*. BMJ, London.

Medical Ethics Committee, BMA (1992) *Guidance on Private Minor Surgery by GPs*. (Guidance note).

Medical Ethics Committee, BMA (1992) *Rights and Responsibilities of Doctors*. BMA, London.

Medical Ethics Committee, BMA (1993) *Medical Ethics Today: its Philosophy and Practice*. BMA, London.

Monopolies and Mergers Commission (1989) *A Report on the Supply of Services of Registered Medical Practitioners in Relation to Advertising*. HMSO, London.

9

Private Medical Records

Importance of medical records

One of the fundamentals of medical practice is the ability to record and make use of information about patients in the interests of their treatment. The ability to record and use such information is a privilege which is subject to certain basic limitations prescribed by law. At one time, patients themselves had no right of access to that information; however, recent legislation has changed all that.

Since November 1987, patients have had a statutory right of access to their health records kept on computer, and from November 1991 they have had limited access to all other health records. Control over information in records prior to these dates depends on ownership of the records.

Ownership of private medical records

The concept of ownership of information is underdeveloped in England and Wales, but at common law the person who 'controls' the records is the person who writes them. Private practitioners who write down information on their own documentary materials therefore control what happens to them (subject to statutory rights of access to information and ethical controls on the disclosure of confidential information) and effectively 'own' those records.

Disposal of private medical records

Unless some agreement to the contrary has been made between the doctor and patient, private medical records belong to the practitioner who creates and controls them rather than the patient who is the subject of those records. The practitioner is therefore at liberty to use and dispose of those records as he sees fit in the interests of his patient. Consideration must, however, be given as to what happens to those records when the practitioner dies. In these circumstances the practitioner's duty of care to his patients dies with him, but the interests of those patients will be best served if the records can be transferred to another doctor who will take responsibility for their care. It is less straightforward if no decision about succession to the practice has been made prior to the doctor's death. Who now owns the records and decides what should be done with them?

If the doctor has left a will, the persons named therein as the executors of his estate or personal representatives have a duty to distribute the doctor's property, including the records of his private medical practice, in accordance with the terms of the will. If no will has been left, ownership of his property will be determined by the statutory rules of intestacy by which the property will devolve first to his surviving next of kin. Persons entitled to the estate can usually apply for letters of administration enabling them to administer that estate. The order is as follows: surviving spouse, children, parents, true brothers and sisters (or their children if they have already died), half brothers and sisters (or their children if they have already died), grandparents, true uncles and aunts (or their children if they have already died), half uncles and aunts (or their children if they have already died).

If the deceased had none of the above, the property devolves first on the Crown, and the Treasury may apply for letters of administration; secondly on the Duchy of Lancaster, whose solicitors may apply for letters of administration; and lastly on the Duchy of Cornwall, whose solicitors may similarly apply. A creditor of the deceased may apply for letters of administration to administer the estate but is not entitled to the estate itself except to the extent of the debt owed to him.

In Scotland the order of succession to a moveable property in intestacy (after the surviving spouse's prior rights have been satisfied) is as follows: the deceased's children and their issue, collaterals (brothers, sisters or their offspring), ascendants (parents etc). Thereafter succession depends on whether there was a surviving spouse. At the end of the day succession ends with the Crown as *ultimus haeres.*

To avoid the problems which arise from intestacy, all private practitioners should have a will and they are advised to leave direct instructions in it as to what should be done with the medical records of the practice in the event of unexpected death. Clearly the well-being of the patients should be of paramount concern and it may be advisable to arrange for the records to be transferred to the safekeeping of another doctor. In the event that no other doctor is found to take over the practice, there is nothing to prevent the doctor or his executors deciding to give the records to the patients to take with them to whichever doctor they now wish to be responsible for their treatment.

In the final analysis there is nothing to prevent the new owners of the records from destroying those records unless there is some possibility of damage to patients being shown to have arisen from such destruction. However, it is possible that in time Parliament may legislate to ensure proper safeguards for the confidentiality of private patients' records and to guarantee as far as possible the continuity of their care.

Concern may be expressed as to what would happen if the person entitled to ownership of the records following the death of a private practitioner decided to misuse them, for example by selling the contents to a newspaper. The new owners of the records must respect the legal duty of confidentiality owed by the original owner of the records to his patient and it should be remembered that private patients might well have a right to sue any person in possession of the records if they were wrongfully to disclose the contents. Once the action had been lodged, an immediate injunction could be applied for to restrain publication. Bearing in mind the difficulties which could arise in such circumstances, the private doctor should always attempt to deal with such matters in his will.

Length of retention of private records

Private practitioners are entirely at liberty to decide how long they wish to keep records of their patients. However it is useful to bear in mind the general guidelines which apply to NHS GP and hospital records. These are as follows:

1   obstetric records: 25 years

2   records relating to children and young people (including vaccination and community health service records): until the patient's 25th birthday or eight years after the last entry if longer

3   records relating to mentally disordered persons within the meaning of the Mental Health Act: 20 years from the date of which, in the opinion of the doctor, the disorder has ceased or diminished to the point where no further care or treatment is necessary (except that such records need only be retained for a minimum of eight years after the death of the patient or in the case of obstetric records, death of the child, but not of the mother)

4   all other personal health records: eight years after the conclusion of treatment.

It should be remembered of course that all records could theoretically be required in litigation virtually without limit of time, and the practitioner should think very carefully before destroying any records which he considers may have a bearing on some future legal case in which he may be involved.

Access to computerized medical records

The Data Protection Act 1984 protects individuals from the misuse of personal information held on computer or some other automated means and requires anyone who controls the contents and use of personal data to register under the Act. Compliance with the Act requires observance of the so-called Data Protection Principles, which require that data:

- be obtained and processed fairly and lawfully
- held for one or more specified and lawful purpose and not be disclosed in any manner incompatible with that purpose
- shall be adequate, relevant and not excessive
- shall be accurate and kept up to date
- shall not be kept longer than is necessary
- shall be accessible to the subject of any data who is entitled to be informed at reasonable intervals that data of which he is the subject is held and where appropriate to have such data corrected or erased
- shall be protected against unauthorized access, alteration, disclosure or destruction of data.

The Data Protection Registrar has the power to execute legal penalties against individuals acting contrary to the above principles. As of May 1986, data subjects have been entitled to compensation if it can be proved they have suffered damage because of loss of data, unauthorized destruction of data, unauthorized disclosure of data or inaccurate personal data (unauthorized destruction in this case means destruction not authorized by the controller of the records in question). As of November 1987, data subjects have had the right to have access to information about them contained in data. The Data Protection (Subject Access Modification) (Health) Order 1987 allows a doctor to whom a request for access is made to withhold parts of the information concerned where he believes that disclosure will cause serious harm to the physical or mental health of the patient. However, no definition is given as to what constitutes serious harm in this context.

Access to Medical Reports Act 1988

The Access to Medical Reports Act 1988 allows individuals to see medical reports written about them for employment and insurance purposes by a doctor who has been responsible for their clinical care. The individual has the following rights under the Act:

- to give or refuse consent for an employer or insurance company to seek a medical report on them

- to see any report after completion by the doctor
- to seek amendment to the report if dissatisfied with it
- to withhold permission for the doctor to send the report to the employer or insurer.

The company (applicant) requesting the report must notify the individual of his rights of access. The doctor must ensure that he has written consent of the individual before the report is written. If he is informed at the time that the application is made that the patient wishes to see the report, he must not send it for 21 days to allow time for the patient to see it. Alternatively, if he receives notification that the patient wishes to see the report after it is written (but before it is despatched to the applicant), he must delay sending the report for 21 days to allow the patient to effect access to it. Once the patient has seen the report it must not be sent until the patient has agreed to its release. If the patient believes there are factual inaccuracies in the report, he may ask for them to be corrected. The doctor is not obliged to make amendments, but if he refuses to amend the report he must agree to attach the patient's statement disputing the information.

In the last resort, consent for the supply of the report can be withheld by the patient. The individual can require access to a copy of the report within six months of it being sent, and for this reason doctors should ensure that accurate dated copies are kept for this period. Where a copy of the report is supplied at the request of the patient, the doctor may make a reasonable charge for the costs of copying it. He cannot charge the patient for simply seeing the report. The doctor has a right to withhold information from an individual seeking access where its release would cause serious harm to that individual's mental or physical health, the health of another person, or where it identifies someone other than a patient or health professional, where that third party has not consented to release of the information identifying him. Failure to comply with the provisions of the Act is a legal offence, but to date no medical practitioners are believed to have suffered any punitive action as a result of non-compliance.

Access to Health Records Act 1990

This Act gives patients, and in certain circumstances other people acting on the patient's behalf, access to manually held health records made after 1 November 1991. 'Health record' is defined as a record of information relating to the physical and mental health of the individual which has been made by or on behalf of the health professional in connection with the care of that person. It applies equally to private and NHS records. The right of access to information is principally for the patient himself if he is capable of understanding.

The patient may also authorize another person in writing to make an application on his behalf. In certain cases defined in the Act other people have the right of access to the patient's records. It is important to note that where the patient has died the patient's personal representative and any person who may have a claim arising out of the patient's death may have a limited right of access to the record relevant to any such claim.

Applications for access must be made in writing to the holder of the records. Once satisfied that the application is correct, the holder must give access to the records within 21 days of the date of application if the record was made within the preceding 40 days. Where the record relates to a period more than 40 days before the application, the holder has 40 days to provide the information. The Act only applies to records made after 1 November 1991, unless, in the opinion of the record-holder, the accessible part of the record is unintelligible without disclosure of information recorded before 1 November 1991. In that case the earlier information must be given to the applicant, unless there is an overriding reason for withholding it.

Where a patient seeks access to records which have not been created within 40 days prior to the request for access, the patient is required to pay a fee to the practitioner, not exceeding the maximum set down in Section 21 of the Data Protection Act 1984 (at present £10). If the applicant wants a copy of such a record or extract, this must be supplied, and a fee may be charged which should not exceed the cost of making the copy and any postage involved.

The applicant is entitled to an explanation of any terms which would not be intelligible to a lay person without explanation. There are certain circumstances where access may be modified or denied:

- where access would cause serious harm to the physical or mental health of the patient or any other individual who could be identified from the information

- where access would involve information provided by or relating to a third party, not being a health professional, who could be identified from that information

- where the relevant part of the health record was made before the Act came into effect on 1 November 1991

- where an application is made by an individual on behalf of the patient because the patient is mentally incapable or has died and the information concerned was given by the patients on the understanding that it would be kept confidential.

If the record-holder grants the applicant restricted access, this would have to be in the form of an extract from the records prepared by the doctor. If a person considers that any part of the health record to which he has had access is inaccurate, he can apply to the doctor to have it corrected. The doctor may either make the necessary amendments or attach a note of the matters the applicant considers inaccurate. The applicant must be supplied with a copy of the correction or note made free of charge. The record-holder is not required to give an explanation of why any part of the record has been withheld. If the holder of the record fails to comply with the Act, however, the applicant can apply for a court order for compliance. Failure to comply with the provisions of the Act is a legal offence. The Secretary of State for Health has powers to determine by regulation what sanctions may be applied against the non-compliant, but has not so far chosen to make use of that power.

The BMA's Medical Ethics Committee has produced guidance notes on the provisions of the Access to Health Records Act and on the Access to Medical Records Act respectively. These are available to members on request.

References and further reading

General Medical Services Committee, BMA (1991) *The Data Protection Act: A Code of Practice for General Medical Practitioners*. BMA, London.

Medical Ethics Committee, BMA (1992) *Rights and Responsibilities of Doctors*. BMA, London.

10

Forms of Business Arrangement

Practising individually or in a group

When setting up in private practice a doctor must decide whether to practise individually or in a group or partnership. GPs will be familiar with both situations. With consultants, the autonomy which they enjoy in their NHS activities militates against group practice, and this is compounded by the prevalence of a system requiring referral to a named specialist. The vast majority of consultants therefore practise individually. However they may come together in various forms of business relationships for limited practical purposes. The group practice 'combine' or partnership is not uncommon among 'tertiary' practitioners, ie those whose services complement those of the surgeon or physician to whom referral of the patient by the primary practitioner (GP) is made in the first instance. These are principally anaesthetists, pathologists and radiologists.

At the time this book was written there were no figures available to indicate how many specialists practise together in partnerships or combines. Surprisingly even the MMC Inquiry into private medical services in 1993 seems not to have provided an answer to this question.

Purchasing an existing practice

Specialists usually seek to set up in private practice at the same time or shortly after their appointment as an NHS consultant. They may fill a vacuum left by their predecessor. If it is a new post, or the predecessor is continuing with his private practice following retirement, it will involve breaking new ground, establishing a client base from scratch, so to speak. Occasionally, however, it may be possible to 'buy' an existing practice, that is to say purchase from a retiring specialist not just equipment, facilities and either the lease or freehold of a property, but also the 'goodwill' attached to an existing client base.

Chambers English Dictionary defines goodwill as 'the established custom or popularity of any business or trade, often appearing as one of its assets, with a marketable money value'. NHS GPs are specifically forbidden to sell the goodwill of an NHS practice. This is because the NHS itself purchased the goodwill of those practices who agreed to join the NHS in 1948 in accordance with a monetary formula negotiated with the profession's representatives at the time. The goodwill of an NHS practice is not therefore within the GP's gift. Accordingly the Medical Practices Committee (MPC) has the power, in accordance with the NHS Act 1977, to withhold approval of any succession to the GP vacancy which actually or implicitly involves a sale of goodwill. This obviously poses some problem when an NHS practitioner with a small private practice wishes to sell the private practice, and he should seek advice on this question from the MPC. There is no prohibition on the sale of goodwill by a specialist or wholly private GP.

Calculating the value of goodwill

Establishing the capital value of a private practice is relatively easy. It will probably not be very substantial, unless a freehold property is involved, in which case the services of an independent valuer will be required. Establishing the value to attach to goodwill is certainly more difficult. Obviously an accountant is the best person to advise on such matters. In one sense a specialist practice may be regarded as a small business but it is an unusual business environment in which, it should be acknowledged, reputation assumes greater importance than in most other businesses.

With most types of business goodwill is calculated on the basis of a multiple of a given year's profit (often twice that amount), but this should not be taken as a hard-and-fast rule. Profits in the year immediately preceding sale may be less than in previous years because the practitioner was 'winding down' his practice or had been less active due to ill health or other reasons. Alternatively the previous year may have been an exceptionally good year in terms of practice activity. It is important to remember that the value to be ascribed to goodwill is entirely negotiable between the parties. The incoming practitioner should obtain from the vendor an accurate index of profit during the preceding few years in order to determine whether the price quoted by the vendor is fair and, if necessary, make a counter offer. The nature of the testimonial or recommendation offered by the outgoing practitioner to existing patients should also be discussed. It may not be considered sufficient simply to hand over the list of names and addresses of the practice clients.

Partnerships

The most common form of business arrangement among medical practitioners is the partnership. This allows individuals to act autonomously, sub-

ject to certain predefined rules requiring the sharing of profit, investment and
liability.

Partnerships are the principal form of relationship between NHS GPs, and
the nature of the agreement need not be substantially different as regards private GPs. NHS GPs will already allow for private practice income to be included in their existing partnership agreements. Income from it will either be
paid directly into the partnership account and profits shared on a predetermined basis (the usual arrangement), or it can be expressly excluded and paid
into the account of the individual partner who earned it (but see Chapter 2 as
regards the 10% abatement provisions).

The specialist 'combine' or consortium

Partnerships are not a practical option for the majority of consultants. However, the partnership 'combine' is an increasingly common feature among anaesthetists and pathologists. This is due to the nature of those specialties.
Whereas patients are referred to individual named surgeons or physicians, the
choice of anaesthetist to assist in any operation required is left up to the surgeon or, on occasion, the private hospital whose surgical facilities are used.
The same will be true of pathology services. As the standard of service offered
by one competent anaesthetist or pathologist is not likely to vary very much
from that offered by another, it is generally considered acceptable for a group
of such individuals to join together in a 'combine' to service the needs of consultants and private hospitals collectively. The 'combine' ensures that there is
always an anaesthetist available whenever the particular surgeon or hospital
wants one.

By forming a partnership, the anaesthetists and pathologists are able to ensure that the supply of work is managed efficiently and profits distributed
fairly while at the same time allowing individuals time off for holidays, educational commitments etc, in accordance with the usual constraints of their
NHS commitments. Obviously the nature of such partnership agreements
will vary but it is understood that many such specialist consortia involve
agreements which provide many of the benefits and safeguards which the
BMA recommends be included in NHS (ie GP) partnerships, including, for
example, remuneration during absence due to sickness.

It is not the purpose of this chapter to offer definitive advice on partnerships. It may be helpful, however, to consider the basic requirements of partnership agreements in broad outline. Authoritative advice on individual
circumstances is best sought from a solicitor and accountant.

Partnerships at will

If a partnership is to prove satisfactory it is essential that the conditions under which it operates should be precisely defined in a properly constituted legal document. This should seek to provide equity for all parties to the agreement. Where parties have not made a specific agreement, a 'partnership at will' can be said to exist. The rights and duties of parties to partnerships, generally including partnerships at will, are laid down in the Partnership Act 1890. In the eyes of the law the existence of a partnership does not depend on the presence of a written agreement but on the conduct of the parties; if the way doctors work together makes them appear to be partners, the law deems them to be partners in fact. Even when a partnership agreement does exist, the Partnership Act is important because it governs the parties relationships with third parties.

Under the rules established by the Partnership Act the liability of the partners is joint and several, ie a patient dissatisfied by the treatment of one partner can sue the whole firm. If such a claim is successful each and every partner is liable for the damages and costs and the property of any one can be taken in execution of the judgement. Alternatively, the patient may sue any one or more of the partners individually.

A partner against whom negligence is proved should indemnify the firm, but may not be in a position to do so. Moreover, even if the patient loses the negligence case and is ordered to pay the partnership's costs, no money may be available to do so. These costs will then fall on all the partners because the partner about whom the complaint is made has done no wrong and he will not be called on to indemnify the firm. Even if costs are awarded against the patient, there is no guarantee that the firm will recover the whole expense it has suffered. The existence of such possibilities reinforces the necessity of belonging to a medical defence organization.

Written partnership agreements

Given the fragility of a partnership at will, and the extremely complex financial structures of modern-day firms, an official deed of partnership is indispensable. The BMA has drawn up a list of essential clauses to be included in any such agreement (not all of which may be necessary in a specialist combine). These are as follows:

- date of document
- practice address
- date of commencement/duration
- practice premises
- income
- attention to firm's affairs

- name and title of firm
- nature of the business
- capital
- expenses
- division of receipt
- tax liability

- engaging/dismissing staff
- holidays/study leave/sabbaticals
- maternity leave
- lengthy incapacity
- restrictive covenant
- arbitration
- accounts

- power to make decisions
- incapacity
- leaving the partnership
- retirement on age grounds
- defence society
- banking
- superannuation

Some of the more important of these basic provisions are explained below. Not all will be relevant to the specialist combine, though they will all apply to the private GP practice.

Partnership capital

The partnership capital includes any property, equipment, stock of drugs, surgery fittings and furniture etc in which there is to be joint ownership, and may also include cash subscribed by the partners as working capital. An incoming partner may expect to purchase a share of the assets at current valuation and contribute towards this capital.

In GP partnerships, a new partner will normally take a reduced share of profits which will increase annually towards parity, normally within three years. Where work and responsibilities are equally shared it is not justifiable for seniority to be recognized by a permanent token difference in shares. For many years it was the accepted principle that partners should own the firm's assets in the same proportion as they enjoy the profits. This meant that normally incoming GP partners would purchase initially a less than equal share in the capital and made further purchases as their share of the profits increased.

Bearing in mind that incoming partners often have the right to increase their initial share of the profits annually, and usually obtain parity in a relatively short time, it is now considered advisable to purchase an equal share immediately or delay purchase until reaching parity, thus avoiding the extra expense of buying the real estate in stages.

In specialist partnerships, immediate parity and equal purchase of shares may be a more practical option.

Expenses

In addition to the rent, rates, heating, lighting and maintenance of the practice premises, the firm as a whole should pay for any practice staff employed, accountancy, stationery, bank charges, practice telephones etc, and such expenses should be paid or allowed before profits are distributed. Other items such as telephones at the partners' homes and car expenses are occasionally paid by the partnership but more usually by the partners individually, this being regarded as more fair. The fact that partnership expenses are paid before distribution of profits means that the partners usually contribute towards such expenses in the same proportion as they share the profit.

Income

Although by no means a hard-and-fast rule, it is usually agreed that the best arrangement is for all fees and professional earnings to form part of the partnership receipts. If partners are entitled to retain some earnings whilst being obliged to share others, it encourages them to apply themselves most diligently to those tasks which are solely beneficial to them.

Attention to the affairs of the firm

The time and attention which the partners are to give to the work of the partnership should be stated, especially if one is at liberty to give less time than the others. In cases where partners are obliged to devote their whole time to the practice, it is also useful to include a stipulation not to engage in any other business requiring their personal attention without the consent of the other partners.

Tax liability

Once a partnership is established, each partner is jointly and severally liable for any income tax on the whole of the net profits of the practice, and any one or all of them could be sued for the whole amount. It is advisable therefore that the partnership agreement should make provision for sufficient monies, as advised by the firm's accountants, to be set aside to meet tax liabilities, preferably in a separate account.

Engaging and dismissing staff

The agreement should state who has responsibility for staff. If a dismissed employee claimed 'unfair dismissal', such a claim would be made against the partnership as a whole. It is therefore advisable that staff employed at the expense of the partnership should be engaged and dismissed only with the consent of all partners. It is also advisable to make provision that any correspondence or documentation relating to staff employment be agreed or vetted by all partners.

Restrictive covenants

Many, if not the majority, of written medical partnership agreements contain what is known as a restrictive covenant. This is a device intended to ensure that an individual who leaves the partnership either voluntarily or involuntarily is prevented from taking the client base with him. A typical restrictive covenant clause will specify that the doctor should not, on leaving the partnership, seek to practise (privately, in this case) in the same specialty within a specified radius of the present practice base, and/or for a specified number of years after his leaving. The law recognizes such covenants as justifiable and proper, provided they are 'reasonable'. It would be unreasonable, for instance, to prohibit the outgoing partner from practising in the area indefinitely, or within an area which would require him to move residence to a town some way distant. Under general law, medical practitioners are entitled to no greater protection than is necessary to preserve their practice.

The restrictive covenant is not usually as important for specialists as for GPs. It is unlikely to be necessary in the case of an anaesthetic combine, for instance, because the large number of partners available on demand renders it unlikely that a surgeon or hospital would seek to go elsewhere, unless there was a choice of 'combines' in that area. The special considerations applying to anaesthetics and pathology are detailed further in Chapter 16.

Business names

Medical partnerships are usually conducted under the true names of individual partners. However, wherever a business is carried on by a partnership and the business name does not consist of the true surnames of all the partners, the Business Names Act 1985 lays an obligation on the partners to disclose the name of each partner and an address within the UK at which documents can be effectively served on that person if necessary. This information must be shown on all business letters, written orders for the supply of goods or services, invoices and receipts and written demands for payment of debts arising in the course of the business, and also by means of a prominent notice displayed in any premises where the business is carried on.

Service companies

We have noted that the partnership is not a practical option for the majority of specialists. A more common form of business arrangement among consultants is the service company. As its name suggests the service company exists for purely functional reasons. Leasing or purchasing a property from which to practice can be expensive when one is only able to devote a limited amount of one's time to private practice. Employing staff to assist with that practice is also expensive, and it is difficult to obtain quality staff on a part-time and sometimes a variable part-time basis. An effective way of dealing with these problems is for a group of consultants to come together to form a company for the limited purpose of leasing or purchasing a property and employing staff on a shared basis.

It is essential that the company remains a non-profit-making concern if it is not to generate tax liabilities for the consultants who have created it. It should therefore be designed to cover its costs and not generate additional revenue. The executive directors of the company are the consultants for whose benefit it exists, and its assets are the property it manages, which—together with the cost of its employees' salaries—use up all of its income. The income is derived from contributions made by the consultants who use those facilities in accordance with a predetermined formula.

While being its directors, the consultants have a contractual relationship with the company as clients using its facilities. Their relationship with each other, however, does not extend beyond being directors and clients of the company. They do not share profits or impinge on each others' professional or financial relationships in the way that a true partnership would do. Sharing the cost of the company's outgoings will vary according to the extent of the use made of them by the individual consultants. How this works in practice will be a matter for the company to determine when it is first established.

Occasionally where service companies have been established to purchase consulting rooms for a group of consultants, other consultants may be permitted to make use of those facilities by renting or leasing them from the company.

The hiring and firing of staff will be effected by collective decisions, the company having liability for all matters relating to the employment of those staff including sick pay, punitive awards for unfair dismissal, redundancy and health and safety at work and for occupiers insurance liability (*see* Chapter 12). Under this arrangement the company is not severally liable for the acts or omissions of individual consultants using the company's facilities in the course of their professional activities.

As with a partnership, the services of an accountant and a solicitor will be required to set up a service company on a proper footing, the expense of which should be shared by those partaking in the arrangement. The service company is a useful device by which consultants can practise in well appointed facilities using trained and experienced staff during the limited time they are able or wish to devote to private practice, without the need for a substantial capital outlay or incurring crippling financial liabilities.

Other companies formed by doctors

Occasionally doctors will come together to form a company which will incur wider responsibilities as regards treatment of patients, ie by offering to provide specific forms of treatment at a private clinic owned by a company. This is not an uncommon arrangement with regard to the provision of fertility services (including abortion), cosmetic surgery, allergy clinics and various forms of alternative therapy, or activities having a medical input such as slimming clinics.

The defence societies have made it clear that they cannot indemnify companies rather than individuals. The following comments by the Medical Defence Union, in its *Benefits of Membership*, should be remembered in this regard:

> 'The Council [of the MDU] will not normally accept responsibility where a claim arises as the result of the engagement of the member in an activity outside the normal range of medical or dental practice, eg where he is the proprietor of a nursing home, a laboratory or a firm providing services to the medical or dental professions.'

There is also a potential ethical difficulty in such arrangements. If the company or an unqualified member of the company derives profit from professional fees earned by a medically qualified member of the company, this could be regarded as fee-splitting (*see* Chapter 8). However, if the whole of the profits of the company are paid to its employees as salary or pension contributions, so that the company shows no profit, this problem should not arise.

The defence organizations also point out, with regard to any form of company in which a medical person is a director, that personal immunity from claims may well be a delusion, because creditors, banks and mortgagers are likely to seek personal guarantees from those directors, and so the idea of limited liability will thereby be nullified.

References and further reading

British Medical Association (1993) *Medical Partnerships in the NHS*. BMA, London.

General Medical Council (1992) *Professional Conduct and Discipline: Fitness to Practice*. GMC, London.

Medical Ethics Committee, BMA (1990) *Information to Companies, Firms and Associations*. (Guidance note).

Medical Ethics Committee, BMA (1990) *Guidelines for Doctors Employed by Private Organizations Providing Clinical Diagnostic or Medical Advisory Services*. (Guidance note).

Medical Defence Union (1986) The Formation of Companies by Doctors. *Journal of the Medical Defence Union*, **Spring**.

Medical Defence Union (1988) Benefits of Membership. MDU, London.

11

Premises and Equipment

Choice of premises

For the private consultant there are essentially three main options as to where to practise privately: in rooms provided in a private or NHS hospital; in 'dedicated' consulting rooms; or in a part of his own home. In choosing, the private consultant will consider his own convenience as well as that of his patients. GPs may practise at home, or in a purpose built surgery or in rented rooms (in London private GPs are also able to practise in consulting rooms in private hospitals).

Consulting in a private hospital

There are several advantages to practising in a private hospital. The standard of accommodation is usually very good, and the rental or lease may include the use of skilled ancillary staff—receptionists, secretaries and nurses—and usually includes most of the basic furniture and equipment. Easy access to on-site pathology and radiology facilities is also a considerable advantage. Payment can sometimes be made on a sessional basis if required.

Increasingly, consultants tend to see their private out-patients at the same private hospital at which they have in-patient admission rights. They and any GPs using private hospital facilities should, however, be mindful of the GMC's rules on financial interests (*see* Chapter 8).

NHS hospital consulting rooms

Use of rooms in NHS hospitals requires formal approval by the hospital authorities. With the advent of NHS Trusts it seems likely that there will be increasing availability of rooms for hire by consultants acting in a private capacity. The more businesslike approach evidenced by Trust managers may lead to the creation of advantageous terms for private practitioners. The use of such facilities by private consultants will be seen as a valuable source of regular additional income.

While junior medical staff are obliged to assist consultants in treating the private patients they have admitted to the hospital, their services and those of nursing and secretarial staff will not be provided free. These will be the subject of a separate contract between the patient and the hospital. Consultants should not ask their NHS secretaries or receptionists to work privately without payment (*see* Chapter 12). Such activities are not part of those individuals' NHS duties, and officially any work which involves assisting the consultant with his private patients should be undertaken outside the hours during which the secretary or receptionist works for the NHS.

'Dedicated' private consulting rooms

The use of such rooms may offer the easiest and best way of practising privately but it is often also the most expensive. Purchasing the freehold of a property will require a substantial capital outlay and is therefore best achieved by practitioners coming together to form a service company (*see* Chapter 10). By this means they may purchase the freehold or lease, together with the necessary equipment, and employ staff used by the practitioners, on a shared basis. Fully equipped consulting rooms can nevertheless be obtained by lease or licence in a number of cities.

The Harley Street medical 'precinct'

In London the area in which private consultants have traditionally practised in this way is centred on Harley Street (*see* Figure 11.1). The words 'Harley Street' conjure up an image of private treatment for the well-off, eg celebrities, aristocrats and foreign dignitaries. For many years Harley Street and its environs (known as the Harley Street medical precinct) was the place to be if you were a full-time private consultant. Despite the persistence of its popular image, however, the importance of Harley Street is undoubtedly diminishing. Indeed many would argue that it is increasingly irrelevant in terms of the domestic market in private healthcare.

However, for the foreign market for private specialist service, Harley Street continues to reap the benefits of its international renown. It has been estimated that about 15% of the total market in private specialist services is made up of foreign nationals and at least two thirds of these are treated in London. Although Laing (1992) claimed that fees for a selection of operations at the beginning of 1992 were considerably higher than in other European coun-

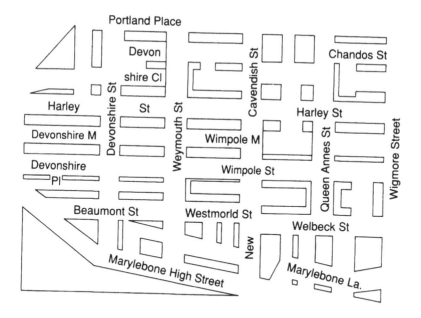

Figure 11.1: The Harley Street Medical precinct.

tries, the continuing popularity of the UK among non-Europeans must say something about the quality of service provided by UK specialists.

One reason for the relative decline of Harley Street in the domestic market is the fact that the area in which medical practice is undertaken in the vicinity of Harley Street is contracting. The owners of many of the properties in the area which were traditionally leased or occupied under licence have recently made over their property for other more profitable uses in the domestic or business fields. The principal 'head landlords', the Crown Estate and the Howard de Walden Estates, have indicated a willingness to preserve the character of the area by maintaining the availability of consulting rooms in the properties under their control. However, smaller landlords are increasingly selling the properties once used for such purposes for domestic development.

The other reason for the demise of Harley Street is the cost of practising in London. Because overheads are high, professional fees are correspondingly higher than in the provinces. However, there is now a general recognition that the quality of service offered is not necessarily superior to that offered by practitioners in other parts of the country. Reputation is a factor used to great effect in the setting of professional fees but in Harley Street it is the reputation of the area which has, for too long perhaps, been used to inflate the level of fees charged for medical services.

Another factor which works to the detriment of Harley Street is the increasing reliance of practitioners on the use of high-technology diagnostic services in out-patient consultations. The consultant leasing rooms in Harley Street is rarely able to afford the best which a consortium of practitioners in the provinces can obtain, and whereas the facilities are available in private and NHS hospitals in London, their use is expensive because of overheads. With the future of many of the Central London hospitals in doubt in the wake of the Tomlinson Report, there may be less choice of such facilities in future and the convenience of the patient can no longer be guaranteed in this respect. Travelling between consulting rooms and hospitals can be a considerable inconvenience in London. It may be less of a problem for a foreign visitor travelling to a hospital by taxi than for the out-of-town resident who has to contend with the problem of parking his own car. Moreover, as consultants lose their NHS base in London hospitals, they may be less able or willing to continue to maintain their private practice base there also.

Lease or licence?

If the private practitioner does decide to obtain rented rooms in the Harley Street area or in similar medical precincts in other major cities, there are two main types of arrangement by which these properties may be let: *lease* and *licence*.

A *lease* confers to the lessee rights prescribed in the terms of the lease. However limited these may be, the existence of the lease confers rights as business tenants under the Landlord and Tenant Act, principally the right to protection against the lease not being renewed without good reason. Exclusion of such rights may only be a term of a lease by order of the Courts. Before such an order is made, the court will need to be satisfied that both parties have been legally advised. A medical practitioner leasing a property acquires business tenant rights to the grant of a new lease on the expiration of this tenancy at a fair rent which will be decided upon by a court if necessary. The relevant legislation lays down set procedures and time limits for the service of notices and counter-notices by both landlord and tenant, and expert advice from both solicitors and surveyors is essential to preserve such rights.

The lease meanwhile confers to the lessor a guaranteed payment of rent and ensures that the property will be occupied and maintained to a degree which the lease prescribes. The agreement may contain covenants requiring the tenants to maintain the property in a good state of repair. However where the premises are occupied by a number of different individuals, as is the case in many of the large properties in the Harley Street area, it is usual for a landlord to agree to be responsible for the upkeep of the fabric of the building in return for service charges being paid for by the tenants.

Normally the terms of a lease enable the lessee to assign the whole of his rights in the property to another person provided that the assignee is respectable and responsible and approved by the landlord. The Landlord and Tenant Act contains provisions enabling application to the court to be made should the landlord's consent be unreasonably withheld. The terms of a lease usually forbid assignment of part only of the property and change of use.

Many leases contain restrictions on the use of the property outside normal business hours (this is the standard arrangement in properties owned by the Howard de Walden and Crown Estates) and forbid the tenants to sleep on the premises (since this might confer residential rights). Leased premises in the Harley Street area usually come fully furnished, but electricity, heating and telephone bills have to be paid for separately.

Many of the properties in the Harley Street area are occupied under *licence* rather than lease. The licensee pays the licensor a licence fee for the privilege of occupying the premises. The business relationship may be formal or informal but, even if included in a written agreement, the licence conveys no lasting rights of occupation. A licence is not a rental and therefore confers no rights under the Landlord and Tenant Act. A licence carries with it no security of tenure and can be terminated on reasonable notice by either party. This may be considered an advantage for the landlord but it does not guarantee continued occupancy of his premises. However it is a common feature of life in Harley Street where renovation of properties by the head landlords frequently leads to them being vacated and reoccupied on a piecemeal basis.

Legal advice should always be sought before entering into any form of tenancy, be it lease or license. The extent of the landlord's interest in the property should be checked. Does he have a freehold interest, for instance, or is he subletting under the terms of his own leasehold interest? The landlord may be a retired medical practitioner or someone with a purely commercial interest in the property. The landlord may also be a service company created by other medical practitioners practising in the same building or elsewhere. A solicitor will check that the landlord has the capacity to grant the proposed tenancy and that it does not contravene the terms of the landlord's interest in the property.

Practising at home

One of the most popular options is to practise from home. This is a familiar situation with a number of GPs who will be acquainted with the tax advantages of combining their home with their practice address. Apart from enabling the practitioner to purchase a large house, practising at home will cut down on travelling costs and will bring entitlement to tax relief in respect of heating, lighting, decor etc. For the practitioner employing his wife as a secretary/practice manager, practising at home may seem the obvious choice. It can, however, lead to resentment at loss of privacy and disruption of the family routine.

Any doctor thinking of practising at home will need to consult his account-ant in order to determine what tax advantages are available, but he must also be aware of the possible disadvantage of the Capital Gains implications should he decide to sell the property. He should also check with his solicitor that there are no restrictions on the use of his property for business purposes, although medical consultation is not usually regarded as 'running a business' in the ordinary sense, as far as property is concerned.

Sharing of premises

The sharing of premises with members of allied professions, including the professional supplementary to medicine, was discouraged for many years by the GMC. This attitude was based on the need to prevent any infringement of the principle of free choice by the patient. Advances in clinical medicine have brought changes in the structure of medical practice, and the present trend is towards closer integration of the various disciplines contributing to patient care.

There is no objection to a surgery being located in a large building such as an office block, provided the doctor's rooms are entirely self-contained so that the patients do not pass through the premises of other tenants on their way to or from the surgery. Doctors may practise from the same building as members of other healthcare professions, if the professional premises are sep-arate and have separate entrances and addresses. The GMC would neverthe-less disparage location of surgeries in hotels or in other buildings which are extensively used by the general public for commercial purposes.

The sharing of premises by general practitioners with specialists is con-sidered acceptable, provided there is no direction of patients, either explicitly or implicitly, which would restrict the patients' potential freedom of choice. This proviso also applies to GPs whose premises are part of a health author-ity-owned health centre, from which members of the professions supplement-ary to medicine also practise.

Stationery

Having established a permanent address, the private practitioner should set about having the necessary business stationery designed and printed. As the cost of stationery is fully tax-allowable there is no need to skimp on quality. Whatever style of letterhead is chosen, letters should clearly show the practi-tioner's name and qualifications, consulting room address and telephone number, together with fax number and telephone number for appointments (if different). In addition to A4 letterheads and continuation sheets, the practitioner will require A5 letters or pads for prescriptions and fee notes or account forms, folders and suitable paper for patient records, compliments slips, appointment cards and formal visiting cards. Many practitioners will carry a supply of stationery with them together with a domiciliary consultation pad when visiting.

Equipment

Office furniture and basic equipment, in addition to secretarial equipment, will be provided in a group facility or a private hospital suite. A consultant or GP setting up on his own will need to provide all this himself. He will need basic furniture—chairs, desk, bookcase, examination couch and professional equipment according to specialty. His secretary will require basic furniture plus filing cabinets and either an electric typewriter or, ideally, a word-processor.

Where the individual is in full-time private practice or undertakes a substantial amount of it, it may be advisable to invest in a computer with which to manage accounts and billing as well as to store and retrieve records (*see* Chapter 13). In addition it is essential to have dictation equipment for both recording and transcribing. Each telephone line used in connection with the practice should be linked to an answerphone with remote control which should be switched on whenever the telephones are not manned. A fax machine can be a considerable bonus, but it is advisable to have one which works independently of the telephone or answerphone. A photocopier is also a considerable boon and inexpensive desktop versions are now available. The busy consultant or GP may also feel the need to invest in a mobile phone. Finally the consulting rooms should be equipped with tea- and coffee-making facilities for the comfort of patients as well as the doctor and his staff.

The Occupiers Liability Acts

Practitioners should be aware of the responsibilities arising from the use of premises for business purposes. The Occupiers Liability Acts of 1957 and 1984 (not applicable in Scotland or Northern Ireland) stipulate what responsibilities are owed to members of the public by occupiers of premises. An 'occupier' in this context is taken to be a person who has some degree of control associated with, and arising from, his presence in, and use of, or activity in, the premises. Wherever doctors occupy premises for medical consultation and treatment they are likely to be responsible under this legislation, and it is essential they are familiar with its provisions.

Responsibility for accidents or other mishaps suffered is variable depending on whether the member of public in question was invited or permitted to be on the premises (eg in the case of a patient) or had not been so invited (eg in the case of a trespasser). Responsibility for the first category of person (hereafter referred to as visitors) involves a duty of care wherein it is 'reasonable to see that the visitor will be reasonably safe in using the premises for the purposes for which he is invited or permitted by the occupier to be there'.

The Unfair Contract Terms Act 1977 limits the extent to which businesses may abrogate their obligations to visitors to their premises by means of disclaimers. It expressly forbids disclaiming of liability for death or injury and goes on to state that liability for other loss or damage can only be contracted out if the term or notice in question is 'reasonable'. However the occupier is under no obligation to a visitor in respect of risks willingly accepted by that visitor.

The Occupiers Liability Act 1957 does provide for a measure of responsibility to the occupiers of premises in respect of people other than visitors. In these cases the occupier may absolve himself from the duty by taking such steps as are reasonable in all circumstances to give warnings of the dangers concerned or to discourage the person from incurring the risk. If the person willingly accepts the risk in question, no duty is owed by virtue of the Act. In view of the above it is of course essential for doctors to be insured against any claim under the Occupiers Liability legislation.

However they should also note the provision of the Employers' Liability (Compulsory Insurance) Act 1969 (not applicable in Northern Ireland). This provides that every employer carrying on any business (this includes a profession) must insure and maintain insurance under an approved policy with an authorised insurer against liability for bodily injury or disease sustained by his employees, and arising out of and in the course of their employment in Great Britain in that business. Failure to insure as above is a criminal offence. The Certificate of Insurance must be displayed in the premises occupied. The Employers Liability (General) Regulations prohibit the inclusion of certain conditions in the insurance policy and fix the amount of cover required.

The Health and Safety at Work etc Act 1974

The Health and Safety at Work etc Act 1974 imposes conditional obligations on employers, the self-employed, business occupiers and workers, any breach of which could result in criminal prosecution. The aims of the Act are stated to be, inter alia, to secure the health, safety and welfare of persons at work and to protect members of the public from risks that might be created by the work activities of others. The following is a summary of the general duties owed by employers to their employees, which the Act requires 'so far as is reasonably practicable':

- to ensure that equipment and working conditions are safe and without risk to health

- to ensure safe use, handling, storage and transport of articles and substances

- to provide information, instruction, training and supervision necessary to ensure the health and safety at work of employees

- to maintain the work premises in a condition that is safe and without risk to health with particular reference to access and egress

- to ensure that facilities and arrangements for employees' welfare at work ensure the provision of a safe working environment.

Except in 'prescribed cases' (eg when an employer employs fewer than five persons), each employer must prepare a written statement of his general policy regarding the health and safety at work of his employees.

The Act also imposes general duties on employers to ensure that their working is safe for and without risk to members of the public. It is a criminal offence to fail to discharge the duties imposed by the Act or its Regulations. One of the most important sets of regulations is the Reporting of Injuries, Diseases and Dangerous Occurrences Regulations 1985. These provide for the compulsory reporting of certain mishaps at work to the enforcing authority including any deaths resulting from an accident at work and any injury or condition arising as specified in the regulations. There is also a duty to report the fact that a person has been incapacitated for more than three consecutive days as a result of an accident at work.

The Control of Substances Hazardous to Health Regulations 1988

Complementary to the Health and Safety at Work etc Act, the Control of Substances Hazardous to Health Regulations 1988 (known hereafter as COSHH) expand and clarify the duties of employers in respect of hazardous substances at work to which employees and others may be exposed. Clinical waste falls within the scope of these regulations. COSHH specifically requires that risk assessments are made of all hazardous substances likely to be encountered as a result of work activity. To ensure that clinical waste does not present a risk to staff and others, suitable control measures must be adopted and this should be included in a written health and safety policy. All employees required to handle and move clinical waste should be adequately trained in safe procedures and in dealing with spillages and other incidents for their area of work. In general practice, principals wil be responsible for ensuring that GP ancillary staff and nursing staff are suitably trained and protected. The employer's clinical waste policy and COSHH assessment will have identified any need for personal protective equipment, and the employer has a further duty under COSHH to ensure that items are provided, used and maintained.

The domestic waste-collection service should not be used for clinical waste. Options for disposal include local authority special collection and disposal services, independent contractors to local hospitals or practitioners who may arrange to take waste by private arrangement to the local hospital incinerator. All contaminated sharps and needles should be placed in a sharps container made to current British standards, and all clinical waste must be clearly identified before it is removed from site for disposal. The Environmental Protection Act 1990 places a duty of care on those who import, produce, carry, keep, treat or dispose of 'controlled waste' to take all measures applicable to prevent unlawful depositing or escape of waste from their control and ensure that it is only transferred to an authorised transporter. The BMA has produced two codes of practice which may be used as training manuals by doctors for their staff to ensure basic awareness and compliance with the legislation. These are *Sterilization of Instruments* (1989) and *The Safe Use and Disposal of Sharps* (1990).

The Ionizing Radiation Regulations 1985

In accordance with the above and the Health and Safety at Work etc Act 1974, regulations were introduced in 1988 – the Ionizing Radiation (Protection of Persons Undergoing Medical Examination or Treatment) Regulations (commonly known as POPUMET) – which laid down a series of requirements to safeguard patients undergoing treatment involving such radiations. These apply to simple X-ray exposures as well as to complex radiotherapy.

The regulations require every exposure of a person to ionizing radiation for a diagnostic or therapeutic purpose to be carried out under the responsibility of a person who is clinically directing such exposure and in accordance with accepted diagnostic or therapeutic practice (regulation 4). Only persons who have received adequate training may direct a medical exposure (regulation 5). Proof of adequate training may be provided by means of a certificate attesting to a person's training (regulation 6). Employers are under an obligation to ensure compliance with the training requirements; to keep a record of the particulars of training of persons they employ and a record of radiation equipment (regulations 7, 8 and 9); they must ensure that expert advice is available to their staff (regulation 10).

The regulations are made enforceable as health and safety regulations under the Health and Safety at Work etc Act 1974, the enforcing authority being the Health and Safety Executive, except for regulation 4 and those aspects of the regulations which relate to the administration of radioactive medicinal products (nuclear medicine), for which the enforcing authority is the Secretary of State (regulation 11).

References and further reading

British Medical Association (1989) *Sterilization of Instruments.* BMA, London.

British Medical Association (1990) *The Safe Use and Disposal of Sharps.* BMA, London.

British United Provident Association (1992) *A Guide to Private Consultant Practice.* BUPA, London.

Elliott G (1992) *'Start as You Mean to Go On': The Consultant's Practical and Financial Guide to Private Practice.* G.K. Elliot, Cheryls Close, London.

General Medical Council (1992) *Professional Conduct and Discipline: Fitness to Practice.* GMC, London.

Laing W (1992) *Healthcare Report: UK Private Specialists' Fees—Is the Price Right?* Norwich Union Healthcare, Norwich.

Medical Ethics Committee, BMA (1993) *Medical Ethics Today: Its Philosophy and Practice.* BMA, London.

Medical Ethics Committee, BMA (1992) *Rights and Responsibilities of Doctors.* BMA, London.

The Control of Substances Hazardous to Health Regulations (1988). S.I. 1988/ 1657. HMSO, London.

12

Employing Staff

Initial considerations

Doctors in general practice will be familiar with factors to be borne in mind when employing staff. For consultants this may be unfamiliar territory. They may have management responsibility for the staff under their supervision in an NHS hospital, but they will have no need to concern themselves with the responsibilities owed to those employees by the employing hospital or health authority. Generally speaking, few private doctors practising individually will feel the need to employ more than one member of staff (usually a secretary who doubles as a receptionist, although occasionally a bookkeeper or practice manager as well). Group practices may find it necessary to employ additional administrative staff together with a nurse or radiographer.

Employment of staff carries with it a number of responsibilities. The law governing employment is dealt with at length in a comprehensive guide written by Norman Ellis (1991). Doctors thinking of employing staff for the first time are advised to obtain a copy.

This chapter is intended to do no more than provide a very brief outline of the rights of employees and to explain what is required of private practitioners as employers.

Statutory rights of employees

The law confers certain employment rights on all employees who work 16 or more hours a week and have two years' continuous service, and employees who work between eight and 16 hours a week and have five years' continuous service. The most important of these are listed in Table 12.1.

Employees working less than eight hours per week have none of these rights. Certain other employment rights apply universally, however, and are not dependent upon the number of hours worked or length of service. These include:

Employment right	Length of service required	
	16 + hours per week	8–16 hours per week
The right to return to work after absence due to pregnancy or maternity leave	2 years' continuous† employment	5 years' continuous† employment
Redundancy pay	2 years' continuous employment	5 years' continuous employment
Unfair dismissal	2 years' continuous employment*	5 years' continuous employment*

† Until October 1994 when TURER regulations enhance rights of employees.

* Except where dismissal on grounds of race (including religion) or sex (including pregnancy as reason for dismissal) when no qualifying period required.

Table 12.1: Statutory rights of employees dependent on hours worked.

Factor affecting work	Employee	Self-employed
Having to do work personally rather than hiring someone to do it	Yes	No
Being told at any time what to do and when and how to do it	Yes	No
Working set hours or a given number per week or month	Yes	No
Risking own money in 'business'	No	Yes
Having final say in how service provided	No	Yes
Having to provide equipment necessary for work (other than small tools)	No	Yes
Having to correct unsatisfactory work in own time and at own expense	No	Yes

Table 12.2: Determining employment status.

- itemized pay statements
- trade union membership
- time off work for trade-union activities and for performance of public duties
- time off for antenatal care
- protected period of notice of redundancy
- the right not to be discriminated against in employment on grounds of sex or race.

Contracts of employment

A contract of employment exists as soon as an employee (whatever their hours) shows his or her acceptance of the employer's terms and conditions of employment by starting work, and both employer and employee are bound by the terms offered and accepted. The initial agreement may be verbal, but the employee working 16 hours or more a week is entitled to written particulars of employment within eight weeks of starting (from November 1993). Those working more than eight hours per week will be so entitled where the employer has more than 20 employees.

The contract should contain details such as the names of the parties to the contract; commencement date and reference to continuity of employment; job title; pay; hours of work; holiday entitlement and holiday pay; sick pay; pensions; notice; and grievance and disciplinary procedures (not essential). It is nevertheless sensible to prepare a comprehensive contract of employment covering these subjects. BMA members can obtain a model contract of employment (for GP practice staff) which should prove suitable, with some amendment, for the private practitioner.

It is always possible to amend a contract of employment; no difficulties should arise provided the employer consults the employee about any changes and provided that the reasons are justifiable. Obviously the employer should seek to obtain the employee's consent to any proposed changes. Consent may be express (verbal or in writing) or implied (ie if the employee continues to work under the contractual terms). If the consent is not forthcoming, however, the employer may still implement the proposed change unilaterally. If this is not to be viewed of a breach of contract on his part, the employer must give adequate notice of the change, show that the change is reasonable of itself, and show that he has acted as a reasonable employer in the manner of consulting the employee about it.

Periods of notice

Employment legislation prescribes the minimum periods of notice that must be given by employer and employee. If the latter has been employed for a month or more, he or she must give the employer at least one week's notice. The employer is obliged to give the employee the following minimum notice:

- for less than two years' employment—one week
- for more than two years' but less than 12 years' employment—one week per year employed
- for 12 years' employment or more—not less than 12 weeks.

Unfair dismissal

Employers must always be mindful of the rights of employees under employment legislation. Industrial tribunals exist to hear complaints by employees who allege their employment rights have been breached and offer legal redress in the form of compensation or reinstatement. Punitive awards can sometimes be made against employers found by tribunals to be in a breach of any of the provisions of this legislation.

Industrial tribunals are principally concerned to hear and determine cases involving allegations of 'unfair dismissal'. An employee has three months in which to complain to a tribunal if he thinks his dismissal was unfair. The law defines the meaning of 'unfair' dismissal. If dismissal is not to be regarded as unfair, the employer must prove that the reason falls within the following categories:

- misconduct
- incapability
- redundancy
- a legal impediment to continuing that employment
- 'some other substantial reason'.

Examples of 'other substantial reasons' might include difficult relationships with other staff, false information on an application form, or reorganization of the business leading to a change in working conditions.

The issue of whether the dismissal was fair or unfair also depends on whether the employer acted reasonably or unreasonably in the manner of instituting dismissal. Dismissal can be deemed to take place not only when the employer terminates the contract of employment with or without notice, but also when the employee walks out in circumstances where the employer's behaviour is held to justify his doing so without notice. This is referred to as 'constructive dismissal'.

It is automatically unfair to dismiss an employee for reasons of pregnancy or childbirth; a dismissal on these grounds may be regarded as a breach of the Sex Discrimination Act, which means that it will be regarded as an unfair dismissal. The Trade Union Reform and Employment Rights Act 1993 established new rights prohibiting dismissal on grounds of pregnancy or childbirth irrespective of length of service.

Sickness

The Statutory Sick Pay (SSP) scheme established a minimum entitlement for sick pay for most employees. The employer is responsible for paying SSP, as an agent for the government, for the first 28 weeks of an employee's sick leave in a tax year. The decision as to whether the employee is eligible rests primarily with the employer (*see* Department of Social Security's leaflet *Employer's Guide to Statutory Sick Pay*, 1985). The employer can then deduct the amount for SSP paid from remittances due to the Inland Revenue by way of employers' NI contributions.

Both full- and part-time employees, including married women paying the reduced NI contributions, are entitled to receive SSP from their employers, provided their earnings are more than a certain amount, although SSP is banded into three rates which vary according to the employee's average weekly earnings. Entitlement does not depend on previous NI contributions or previous service with the employer. After 28 weeks' sickness absence, employees still on sick leave will only qualify for state sickness benefit if they have paid the full rate of NI contributions for the qualifying period.

Maternity

The employer must pay Statutory Maternity Pay (SMP) to a pregnant employee for up to a maximum of 18 weeks if she has 26 weeks' continuous employment with that employer prior to the 15th week of pregnancy, and weekly earnings above the lower NI limit (*see* the Department of Social Security's leaflet *Employer's Guide to Statutory Maternity Pay*, 1985). SMP is payable in two rates, the higher rate being payable after two years' continuous employment with that employer for employees working over 16 hours a week, and five years' continuous employment for employees working between eight and 16 hours per week. There is no entitlement for employees who work less than eight hours per week.

The Trade Union Reform and Employment Rights Act 1993 requires that as from October 1994 all pregnant employees will be entitled to 14 weeks' unpaid maternity leave irrespective of length of service or number of hours worked, and have the right to return to work. The maximum period of maternity leave an employee is entitled to take is 40 weeks. However, it should be noted that legislation does not require the employer to pay an employee on maternity leave any amount in excess of the total of 18 weeks' SMP. The Government is expected to announce new regulations amending the SMP scheme during 1994.

Prior to October 1994 any woman who qualifies for maternity leave and who has been continuously employed by that employer for at least two years is entitled to return either to her previous job, or to other suitable work if it is not 'reasonably practicable' for her employer to offer her previous job back. However, if the employer has five employees or fewer, the woman cannot claim unfair dismissal if the employer finds it impracticable to take her back.

Other relevant factors

Almost all responsible employers will make provision for holiday pay, even though employment legislation does not require any employer to pay either a full-time or part-time employee during holiday periods.

As we have seen, the part-time employee takes longer to acquire many rights of employment protection than the full-time employee. Another point to bear in mind when it comes to employing part-timers is that they are sometimes paid at an hourly rate lower than that of full-time employees and employers normally only pay overtime rates to part-timers if they work beyond the full-time working week.

Employment of NHS secretaries

NHS consultants have traditionally asked their NHS secretaries to assist them with the administration of their private practice and category 2 work. This is an area in which particular care should be taken. The position of an NHS-employed secretary differs as between the consultant's private practice and category 2 work respectively. It is accepted that NHS staff should assist the consultant with category 2 work. Such assistance will form part of their normal employment duties for which they will receive no extra remuneration, assuming it takes place during that employee's normal contracted hours. If the employed secretary is asked to work outside normal hours such work should be remunerated, as should assistance with administrative work relating to the consultant's private practice. If such assistance is of an ad hoc nature, the secretary may be regarded as undertaking such work in a self-employed capacity and be responsible for declaring any payments received for tax purposes.

If, however, the consultant employs his NHS secretary in respect of a regular number of hours, representing a substantial commitment outside her normal NHS employment, there is a possibility that the Inland Revenue will regard this arrangement as an employer–employee or 'master and servant' situation. In such cases, the consultant may have to deduct employees' tax and national insurance, if payments made exceed the NI threshold, and become liable for employers' tax and NI contributions.

Employee or self employed?

The criteria by which the Inland Revenue decide whether a person is employed or self-employed for tax and NI purposes are reproduced in a free leaflet (*Employed or Self-Employed*) published by HM Inland Revenue. These are summarized in Table 12.2.

From this it should be clear that a secretary who works irregularly from home using her own typewriter is more likely to be regarded as self-employed than if she works in a private capacity for a consultant at an NHS hospital where she also happens to be responsible to that consultant as an NHS employee.

An alternative worth considering, if the administration work involved in private practice is regular and considerable, is for the consultant to approach the hospital and contract with them to use the services of a secretary or secretaries on payment of appropriate consideration to the hospital. This would involve the hospital making such secretarial assistance part of the secretaries' contactual duties, but it would absolve the consultant of any responsibility for paying the secretaries' tax and national insurance. If this proves too expensive or impractical, or if the hospital is simply unwilling to hire out secretarial employees for such purposes, the only alternative is for the consultant to employ a part-time secretary and accept that he will have to bear the responsibilities of an employer.

Tax and National Insurance

But what are the responsibilities of an employer vis-à-vis tax and national insurance? Once the practitioner is satisfied that the person working for him is an employee and not self-employed, he has to inform the tax office of the date the employee started working for him; work out the tax and NI contributions due each pay day; pay this over to the tax accounts office each month; and tell the tax office at the end of the year how much the employee has earned and how much tax and national insurance the practitioner has deducted.

When first taking on an employee, the practitioner should telephone the tax office which deals with his tax affairs and ask them for the name of the appropriate PAYE office, as it may be a different one from his own. Alternatively he should fill in the form provided for the purpose in free tax leaflet IR53 and send it to his tax office for onward transmission to the appropriate PAYE office.

The tax office will send him an information pack, the *Employer's Basic Guide to PAYE*. This guide consists of a series of cards (the P8 cards) containing detailed information for operating PAYE together with a new employer's starter pack containing relevant instructions, tables and forms for PAYE and NI contributions.

An employer has to deduct tax from all employees who are paid more than a certain rate (determined annually by the Chancellor, details of which are available from the local tax office). Employer's and employee's NI contributions also have to be paid if the employee's earnings exceed a different specified amount each week or month (details of which are available from the local tax or DSS office). Tax and NI contributions must also be deducted from SSP or SMP paid by the employer exactly as if they were earnings.

The practitioner should ask his employee for his P45 and National Insurance number. The P45 is a leaving certificate given by the last employer. The practitioner should send part of it to the tax office and keep the remainder. If the employee does not have a P45, the practitioner should provide the employee with a starting certificate (P46) to sign. Normally the employer completes the rest of the P46 and sends it to the tax office.

Working out what tax and NI to deduct

To work out the employee's tax and NI contributions, the employer will need the relevant PAYE code (for each employee), tax and NI contribution tables and a deductions working-sheet for each employee. A PAYE code is usually a number and a letter. It represents the amount of the employee's tax allowances, ie tax-free pay for the year. It is used with the tax tables to find out how much pay is tax free each pay day. The employee's tax code will be shown on his P45. If he does not have a P45, the Inland Revenue starter pack will explain what to do.

Tax tables come in two parts. First there are the free pay tables. By looking up the employee's tax code, the employer can determine how much of his employee's pay is tax-free each month. He should deduct the total of the tax-free pay from the earnings leaving the taxable pay and then consult the taxable pay tables to see how much tax is due. The NIC tables will show how much

NIC should be paid on the money the employee earns that week or month. NICs are calculated separately on the pay for each week or month but PAYE is usually worked out on the running total of pay in the year up to each pay day.

Every month the employer should send all the tax he has deducted and all the NICs payable to the accounts office with the pay-slips provided. After the month has ended he is allowed 14 days to send in these payments.

If the practitioner is starting up in business and has not yet been sent pay-slips from his accounts office he should keep any tax and NI contributions deducted from his employees until these pay-slips arrive. As soon as they arrive the full amount should be despatched to the accounts office with the pay-slips. After that the practitioner should use the pay-slips to send tax and NI contributions to the accounts office within 14 days of the end of each month.

If the employee should leave, the employer should provide a P45 (leaving certificate) with the totals of the employee's pay and tax from the deductions working-sheet. The P45 is in three parts. Part 1 is sent to the tax office and parts 2 and 3 are handed to the employee to give to his or her next employer so that the right amount of tax can be deducted in future.

At the end of the year the employer must complete a summary for each employee for whom he has used a deductions working sheet during the year. He must provide a copy of this to all employees still with him. He should then record all the details on one statement and send this to the tax office. All the instructions, tables and forms needed to operate PAYE and NI contributions are contained in the new starter pack. However the local tax office will be able to help with enquiries and there are also tax enquiry centres which have been set up especially to deal with questions about PAYE. The address of the nearest office can be found in the phone book under 'Inland Revenue'.

Employment of spouses

Since the introduction of independent taxation wives are treated as separate individuals for tax purposes. A number of private practitioners employ their wives as secretaries/receptionists/bookkeepers. If the wife's duties can be substantiated, the salary the practitioner pays her will be allowed against his fee income for tax purposes. However, it should be noted that the Inland Revenue generally view such claims with suspicion. The practitioner's wife will be allowed up to the ceiling of a single person's tax allowance. In 1992/93 the threshold for PAYE consisted of a monthly salary of £287 and the threshold for NI contributions was £234.

In general, for any claim to succeed the following criteria must be satisfied: (1) the salary must actually be paid to the spouse and not exist on paper only, and (2) the salary must appear reasonable having regard to the services rendered or duties undertaken.

Pension contributions for an employed spouse may also be allowed, but exceptionally high payments will certainly attract investigation by the Inland Revenue.

Where the practitioner's wife is herself a qualified doctor there is great scope for tax savings if both work together as partners in the same practice. As always, the advice of an accountant would be helpful in establishing the most tax-effective way of treating such employment.

References and further reading

Advisory Conciliation and Arbitration Service (1993) *Employing People*. ACAS, London.

Department of Social Security (1985) *Employers' Guide to Statutory Maternity Pay. Leaflet no. NI228.*

Department of Social Security (1985) *Employer's Guide to Statutory Sick Pay. Leaflet no. NI227.*

Ellis N (1993) *Employing Staff, 5th edn.* BMJ, London.

HM Inland Revenue (1992) *Employed or Self-Employed. Leaflet IR56/NI39.*

HM Inland Revenue (1992) *Employers' Basic Guide to PAYE. Leaflet IR53.*

13

Practice Accounts and Collection of Fees

Accounting procedure

Precise bookkeeping and accounts are essential to the success of any small business, and private medical practice is no exception. Without proper accounts the business of the practice cannot be managed efficiently, economically or tax-effectively. Practices with a large turnover may find it necessary and desirable to employ a bookkeeper. A single-handed practitioner with a modest turnover may prefer to delegate that responsibility to his secretary or spouse or even manage his accounts personally. The rudiments of bookkeeping are easily explained, but the advice of a bank manager or accountant may help to set the newly established practitioner off on the right footing.

One of the first acts of the practitioner setting up in private practice for the first time should be to open a practice bank account into which he will pay fees received and from which he will pay the expenses of running his practice. A paying-in book provided for the purpose should be used for crediting the account with fees received. Regular expenses should be paid where possible by direct debit from the account. Private withdrawals from the practice account should be transferred to the practitioner's personal account and the transaction recorded to enable the practitioner's accountant to keep track of where the money has gone at a later date. By ensuring that all practice business is transacted via the single account the practitioner will ensure that his accountant has an accurate record of income and expenditure for the purposes of assessing the practitioner's tax liability.

The practitioner should ensure that sufficient money is set aside on a regular basis to cover anticipated tax liability. To facilitate this he should open a separate interest-bearing tax reserve account at a bank or building society in which to set aside such monies. During the first year of practice, 20% of fee income should be sufficient to cover the initial tax liability. Keeping track of income and expenditure by means of a monthly budgetary statement, the practitioner will soon find out whether 20% will be enough and whether to adjust the figure upwards as necessary.

A regular cash-flow statement is a useful device with which to keep abreast of the cash-flow difficulties which beset all small businesses from time to time. It will serve to alert the practitioner to problems of rapidly rising or falling income, and serve as a useful record for a bank manager or lender if an urgent overdraft or loan is required. As the business progresses it will be possible for the practitioner or his staff to prepare accurate cash-flow forecasts which will be invaluable to him both as an essential management tool and to assist in forward planning.

Fee records

The appointments diary is the simplest and most immediate record of work carried out. It should record not just the date and other details of consultations, investigations and operations undertaken, but also the fees due in respect of the patients named. If, as often happens, the appointments book contains alterations, a separate day-book or patient ledger is advisable. Staff should transfer the details from the appointments diary to the patient ledger at regular intervals. The ledger will serve as a permanent record of fees billed, fees received and fees outstanding. To assist in keeping the patient ledger details accurate, it is suggested that a daily list of patients be drawn up from the appointments diary on which the practitioner can transcribe details of the treatment undertaken and the appropriate fee. Once the details have been transferred from this daily sheet on to the patient ledger the sheet can be filed. The sheets can provide the practitioner's staff with the information necessary to prepare the monthly budgetary statement referred to earlier.

Billing and collection of fees

The number of each invoice sent out to patients should be entered against the patient's name in the patient ledger and copies of the invoices as they are issued filed in chronological order in an 'unpaid' file. As accounts are paid the invoice can then be transferred to a 'paid' file. The details of any credit notes should be suitably transcribed in the patient ledger. The same process should be applied to expenses paid out, with unpaid and paid invoice files supported by cheque counterfoils.

Opinion differs as to how soon to send bills to patients seen. It is not considered unreasonable to issue a bill within seven days after the first consultation, with a reminder 21 days later if the account is not yet settled. Difficulties with overseas patients are best avoided by insisting on payment at the time of the consultation.

A practice of sufficient size may keep such records in a more formal sales ledger, from which balances of debtors might be extracted at frequent intervals.

The invoice should be precise and factual, containing no more than the following details:

- date

- patient's name and address

- date of consultation (or date of admission to hospital and discharge, if appropriate)

- name of hospital the patient is admitted to (if appropriate)

- name of surgical or investigative procedure (if appropriate)

- fee.

Petty cash

The practitioner should avoid using fee income to cover minor practice disbursements as this will make accounting more difficult later. Petty cash should be dealt with properly using an imprest system. This involves establishing an initial cash float from the practice account. Every item purchased using this money should be receipted and at any one time the sum of cash and receipts should add up to the total of the original cash float. Sums equivalent to the receipts should be drawn from the practice account each month to replace the amounts expended and bring the float back to its original figure.

The systematic and accurate recording of petty cash transactions is essential in any well managed business. Although the amounts may not be substantial in total, imperfect control of petty cash can create significant accounting problems.

Processing fees and expenses

Cheques for cash received in payment of fees should be paid into the practice account via the paying-in book, with the name of the payee being written on both the paying-in slip and the stub of the paying-in book. Records should be made of the payment and the date on which it was received in both the patient ledger account and in the receipts side of the practice cash-book. It often transpires that insured patients will contact the practitioner to enquire if payments have been received from the patient's health insurer to cover the cost of treatment carried out. Such enquiries can be answered readily by consulting the patient ledger. As regards expenses, a separate book can be kept equivalent to the patient ledger detailing expenses. This should be handed with the relevant receipts to the accountant at the end of each year.

Direct settlement

The traditional method of settling bills covered by health insurance is for the patient to pay and claim reimbursement from the insurer, either before or after settlement. In recent years a number of health insurers have, as we have seen, instituted a system of direct settlement whereby they offer to pay the doctor directly without patient involvement. As has been noted, one reason for this is a desire to exercise greater control over fees. Patients are more likely than insurers to settle in full the bills of specialists whom the insurers might suspect of charging excessive amounts. Direct settlement facilitates direct contact between the insurers and specialists, enabling the former to exert pressure on the latter should they consider them to be charging too much. This is not to say that direct settlement has ruled out higher fees. Nor has it prevented patients occasionally being left like 'piggy in the middle', facing an additional bill representative of the shortfall between the specialist's fees and what the insurer is prepared to reimburse. However, it has had the effect of identifying and marginalizing those whom the insurers consider to be guilty of overcharging.

In general specialists have welcomed direct settlement as a means of speeding up payment and obviating the difficulties of chasing patients for monies owed. It has, nevertheless, brought its share of problems to a number of practitioners. In the case of BUPA, this was compounded by the introduction of a system of payment whereby amounts in respect of more than one subscriber treated by a particular specialist would be paid in bulk. This system also provides for virement of payments made to individual practitioners. Some specialists complained, for instance, that overpayments made in respect of one patient were made good at a later date by deducting an equivalent amount from the bill due in respect of a completely different patient.

Although BUPA provides computer-generated 'provider statements' containing all the necessary information regarding any such adjustments made, the havoc which this can cause to practice accounts when something goes wrong can easily be imagined. Having rectified some of the problems which appeared when this system of payment was first introduced BUPA maintain that only a couple of hundred consultants have so far chosen to opt out of the system of direct settlement.

Use of new technology

There can be no doubt that new technology can be a boon for the small businessman. Office administration and management of accounts can be transformed by investment in and usage of appropriate hardware and software. Apart from simple identification data, a computer can be used to record details of consultation dates, diagnoses, tests, surgical procedures and follow-up treatment. It can also be used to prepare bills, monitor unpaid bills and issue reminders, record income and expenditure, and offer, at a glance, the up-to-date financial situation of the practice. Packages which offer such benefits can be obtained 'off the shelf' for use on simple word-processors. However more advanced databases permit a much wider use of administrative functions including the sorting of records according to different criteria.

The drawback as far as new technology is concerned is that you only get out what you put in. Successful use of data is dependent on accurate entry. This may involve a good deal of the practitioner's or staff's time initially, together with a good deal of perseverance. This generates a cost factor which should be taken into account when considering whether to purchase an appropriate computer package.

There are a limited number of companies specializing in packages for the private practitioner, though a good many suppliers in the enormous GP computer market may well be able to offer a custom-built package for an appropriate consideration. Some enthusiasts may wish to design their own packages. For those wishing to organize payroll data in this way, the Inland Revenue will provide some helpful 'computer user notes'. These can be obtained by writing to the Inland Revenue, Comben House, Farriers Way, Bootle, Merseyside, L69 9EU.

Processing insurance claim forms

Medical health insurance claim forms have to be signed or validated either by the consultant who has carried out the treatment or the patient's GP, according to the rules of that particular insurance scheme. In completing the account of treatment carried out, specialists should describe the diagnosis and investigative procedures or operations in full. Most insurers use a coding system for operations based on the OPCS 4 classification of operations (with elements of the Korner codings for consultations and diagnostic procedures). With minor differences of interpretation these codes are common to the BUPA and PPP schedules and the BMA Guidelines.

When received, the claims are assessed by non-medically qualified clerks. Disputes over fees and what the procedure involves can be lessened if the fullest possible information is supplied. Specialists should always keep copies of completed forms and, where the claim is sent directly to the insurer, are advised to send a copy to the patient for information. It is also important to keep some separate record of the reference number given to the claim by the insurer (it could, for instance, be written in the patient ledger book).

Problems of recovery

It is a fact of life for any business that there will sometimes be problems with unpaid bills. The reasons for non-payment of bills for private medical treatment are many and various. If the patient is responsible for paying his own bill, it could be that he is financially embarrassed or simply forgetful; that he disputes the appropriateness of the bill or is refusing to pay because he is dissatisfied with the outcome of the treatment; or it could simply be that he is dishonestly seeking to avoid payment altogether. If the patient is covered by health insurance, delays or failure to pay bills for consultations and treatment may be due, as is often the case, to a dispute between the patient and insurer over the amount due. It could be that the insurer feels the fee charged is too high and will not agree to pay it or fully reimburse the patient if he pays it; or it could be the insurer refuses to pay for the treatment because it is not covered by the patient's policy, either because it is excluded for one reason or another or because the patient has exceeded his benefit limit; or it could be because the treatment has been carried out by a doctor whom that particular insurer will not recognize as a specialist.

Legal action

Private treatment is, as we have seen, based on a contract between the patient and the doctor, whatever the nature of the payment arrangements. Even if, in the practitioner's estimation, it is the insurer who has failed to honour a pledge to the patient to pay the specialist's fee, or has in some other respect reneged on agreements entered into, the legal remedy does not lie with the insurer but with the patient. It is therefore the patient against whom the doctor must pursue the claim in a small-claims court to recover the money owing. If the patient has been let down by the insurer, the practitioner may feel reluctant to do so and will no doubt choose to seek redress from the insurers by writing to them to ask them to make good their promise to the subscriber.

However, if it is simply a question of a shortfall between the doctor's fee and what the insurer will charge, the doctor may well have forewarned the patient, as he is advised to do by the BMA, either verbally or in writing. The practitioner may then feel there is no impediment, moral or otherwise, to pursuing the claim against the patient in the courts. There may, however, be other impediments. Physicians who are members or fellows of the Royal College of Physicians will be aware that certain arcane rules forbid them from taking legal action to recover fees from patients. The reason for this was no doubt a concern for the public image of the profession, coupled with a desire to discourage venality amongst its members. In practice, however, this ruling may prove a headache for physicians who have been fleeced by unscrupulous or dishonest patients.

Debt collection

An alternative to legal action, popular among many practitioners, is to employ a commercial debt-collecting agency to pursue the defaulter. Such agencies act on a 'no win, no fee' basis: that is, if they do not succeed in recovering the fee from the patient, they will not charge the doctor for their services. Another option is simply to transfer the debt to a third party, including, for instance, a debt collecting agency, for a consideration less than the amount of the debt itself. The third party may well have fewer qualms about the methods employed to recover the debt. Practitioners who resort to such methods presumably do so out of a desire to wash their hands of the sordid business of pursuing debtors.

If the practitioner decides to take legal action he may employ his solicitor to write to the patient informing him of the impending legal action and penalties involved. This will involve additional expense.

There are particular areas of private practice where failure to pay bills is becoming commonplace. Psychiatrists, for instance, often complain about non-payment for consultations and often find that they have no option but to refuse to allow regular consultations to continue unless the bill is paid. As far as the health insurers are concerned the application of 'managed care' will rule out many of the present difficulties with payment for psychiatric treatment.

Patients from overseas who are neither resident or domiciled in the UK are notorious for failing to pay bills for private treatment even when, as is often the case, their embassy may have agreed to be responsible for payment. In the event that the patient leaves the country without paying and with no declared intention of returning, the practitioner cannot entertain much hope of receiving payment. His only option is to write to the embassy of the country in which the patient is normally resident to enlist their help in obtaining payment. To avoid this eventuality, many private practitioners treating patients from abroad insist on payment at the time of consultation.

Preventative measures

The practitioner should take whatever precautions he feels appropriate to ensure that his patient will be in a position to meet his bill. He should enquire beforehand if the patient is covered by health insurance, and if the answer is yes, he should question the patient further as to the type and extent of the policy in question. He should then advise the patient of the likely cost of treatment and encourage him to double check with his insurer that such costs will be met or reimbursed.

If the patient is not insured the practitioner will use his judgement, knowing that the majority will pay their bills without demur but that some will, for a variety of reasons, prove reluctant to settle their account. If the circumstances militate against recovery of the money by any of the means listed above the practitioner may have no option but to list it as a bad debt. Proper and timely accounting and monitoring of cash flow should ensure that the number of such debts does not increase to an unacceptable level, though medical practitioners are usually spared the worst effects experienced by other small businesses.

References and further reading

British United Provident Association (1992) *A Guide to Private Consultant Practice*. BUPA, London.

Elliot G K (1992) *'Start as you Mean to go on': The Consultant's Practical and Financial Guide to Private Practice*. G.K. Elliot, Cheryls Close, London.

Medical Ethics Committee, BMA (1992) *Rights and Responsibilities of Doctors*. BMA, London.

14

Taxation

The difference between Schedules D and E

Almost all doctors working in the private sector do so as independent contractors. As such their income from private practice falls to be assessed for taxation under Schedule D, the schedule applicable to the self-employed, rather than Schedule E, the schedule applicable to employed earners.

The income of NHS general practitioners is also assessed under Schedule D. Because their NHS income is derived from a multitude of sources (eg capitation payments, item of service fees and miscellaneous allowances), the computation of their accounts is a complex matter. Almost all GPs therefore employ an accountant to do their books and prepare their accounts for Inland Revenue inspection. Income from any non-NHS work they undertake may be regarded either as practice income or as income earned by the partner who did the work. Almost all non-NHS work undertaken by GPs will be assessed under Schedule D. The only exceptions will be work involved in part-time appointments which are regarded by the Inland Revenue as an 'office' or employment. Company doctor and school medical officer posts may fall into this category, depending to some degree on the nature of the engagement.

The position of wholly private GPs and wholly private consultants is identical to that of NHS GPs in this regard, although their accounts will be less complex to prepare because their income is entirely fee-based, and does not have to take account of the multitude of NHS allowances.

For NHS consultants taking up private practice for the first time, accounts and taxation will seem bewildering and incomprehensible. NHS consultant posts are salaried appointments, the income from which will have been taxed hitherto on a pay as you earn (PAYE) basis under Schedule E, with the hospital deducting tax and national insurance at source before remitting the balance to their consultant employee. For private practice purposes the consultant will be treated as a self-employed person who will be required to produce details of his annual income and expenditure for submission to the Inland Revenue so that his income tax and national insurance liability can be assessed. To this end he will have to complete an annual tax return and set aside money to pay the amount of tax for which he will be assessed to be liable at the due date. Fortunately an accountant will assume most of the burden of managing his tax affairs, particularly the preparation of accounts and any negotiations with the Inland Revenue which may be required. It is an accountant's job to ensure that his client is able to retain the maximum amount of his income by ensuring that every available tax allowance is taken into account. Practitioners would be well advised to employ an accountant who is familiar with the intricacies of medical practice. It is worth asking a prospective accountant whether he has any such experience and how many medical clients he looks after.

All doctors thinking of setting up in private practice are advised to seek advice (either from an accountant or their bank manager) as to the best way in which to manage their accounts from the outset and to obtain the services of an accountant to manage their tax affairs. A number of consultants and GPs may prefer to manage such matters for themselves. Errors in preparing accounts can be costly, however, and medical practitioners are generally ill equipped to deal with problems arising in relation to tax, and may well find themselves at a disadvantage in making representations to the Inland Revenue when appealing against an adverse assessment. With these caveats in mind this chapter will attempt to outline the essential features of taxation applicable to private practice income.

Income, expenses and allowances

Taxable income for these purposes can be described as the excess of income over deductible expenses and capital allowances during the requisite tax year. So what are deductible expenses? Expenses which are tax-deductible under Schedule D are those said to be 'wholly and exclusively' incurred in professional activities. However, a proportion of expenses not 'wholly and exclusively' incurred can also be allowed (*see* Figure 14.1). For Schedule E purposes expenses can only be allowed if they are 'wholly, exclusively *and necessarily* incurred' in performance of the duties of an office or employment. This means that the expense, to be allowed, must be one which each and every holder of that office (eg consultants as a class of employee) is liable to incur, and must be essential to the performance of that office or employment. Such expenses should be claimed from the employer for whom the work is undertaken. The Inland Revenue will not allow any mixing of Schedule E and Schedule D expenses. Because Schedule D expenses need not be 'necessarily' incurred, the private practitioner may often permit himself the luxury of purchasing the most expensive items of equipment and consumables and receive the full tax benefit. As regards motor expenses, only the proportion assessed as being due to business use will be allowed. It is therefore essential to maintain accurate records of business as opposed to domestic mileage. It is also advisable to record all expenses such as petrol, repairs/servicing, tax and insurance so that the Revenue can determine the percentage due to business as opposed to private usage.

When a consultant employed under an NHS contract uses his car for NHS purposes he will already be in receipt of a proportion of motor expenses, some of which will be subject to PAYE. These will be offset by the Inland Revenue in the assessment of expenses from private use allowable under Schedule D.

Expenditure on medical supplies is allowable as a deduction in the accounting period in which it is incurred, but the tax authorities may expect any stock in hand at the beginning and end of the period to be taken into account.

As regards premises, expenditure such as rent, rates and repairs can be allowed against tax in proportion to that part of it where the practice is carried out. It will not therefore include any part which relates wholly to a private residence, and as regards a part of it relating both to the business and a residence (eg repairs to the roof), only a suitable proportion of expenditure is allowed.

Staff costs allowable against tax will include the salaries and employers' NI contributions and private pension scheme contributions in respect of any persons employed by the practice. It is even possible to claim an appropriate proportion of costs of wages and NI contributions of cleaners or domestic help in some cases. (As regards salaries of employed spouses, *see* Chapter 12.)

A doctor who holds a NHS hospital appointment cannot claim tax relief for travel from his consulting rooms (or home) to the NHS hospital. However, mileage costs relating to his private practice can be allowed. When a percentage of car expenses is agreed with the Revenue it is important that the doctor reviews this each year to see if it is still appropriate; otherwise his tax office might not only raise additional assessments for the current year, but might also apply them to up to six years' previous assessments to which interest would be added.

Bank interest on overdrafts or loans entirely for practice purposes including purchase of premises together with hire purchase commitments can also be allowed against tax. A full list of items allowable, together with the percentage normally applied, is shown in Table 14.1.

Capital allowances

A certain amount of tax relief is available in respect of capital expenditure in the form of capital allowances. Payment of capital allowances for such things as equipment, furniture or car purchase involve consideration of a depreciation factor. As their value is reduced annually by depreciation so the value of the capital allowance reduces accordingly. The amount allowable for writing down against the value of the item is normally 25%, eg if a piece of medical equipment cost £1000 in, say, November 1992, the writing down allowance

Expenses/capital allowance	Maximum proportions normally allowed
Accountancy and other professional charges	100% relating to private practice business
Bad debts	100% of amount of actual or estimated bad debts
Capital items, fixtures, fittings and equipment	25% of cost allowed to be written down each year
Cars	£3000 or 25% written down allowance on cost or written down value annually (whichever is the less). Restricted by the same proportion as for motor expenses.
Claims for professional negligence	100% of any excess not covered by insurance
Conference expenses	100% where directly concerned with private practice work and not paid for by NHS allowances (any holiday element regarded as incidental)
Hire purchase/other interest payments	100% where concerned with purchase of equipment for practice. For car purchase the proportion related to business only.
Laundry, cleaning, replacement of white coats	100%
Medical journals, periodicals etc	100% subject to capital allowance for large expenditure
Medical supplies	100%
Motor expenses	Proportion of cost attributable to private practice business (may apply to more than one car)
Other travelling expenses including taxis, train fares etc	100% in connection with practice business (no allowance for home to practice travel)
Permanent health (sickness) insurance premiums	None (unless the practitioner is over 60 years of age)
Printing, stationery and postage	100%
Professional subscriptions	100% where connected with private practice and not claimed against Schedule E income
Protective (but not everyday) clothing	100%
Rental of consulting rooms and facilities	100%
Repairs and renewal of instruments	100%
Residence expenses	Proportion of total heat, light, rates, repairs, insurance expenses etc in relation to practice area occupied
Salary paid to spouse or staff	Dependent on duties and qualifications of spouse or assistant
Secretarial assistance, staff salaries and assistant fees	100%
Telephone	100% at consulting rooms. Proportion of home telephone usage attributable to business (less any NHS reimbursement)

Table 14.1: Expenses allowed under Schedule D (as applicable during 1992–93).

in the first year would be 25% of £1000 ie £250, in the second year a further writing down allowance of 25% of £750 (£1000-£250) will be available, and so on, on a reducing basis until the equipment is sold. With motor cars the figures allowed are £3000 or 25% of the reducing balance (whichever is the less). For assets other than cars a temporary 40% allowance can be claimed when the asset was bought between 1st November 1991 and 31st October 1993.

Earnings basis

Profits are normally calculated on an earnings basis, ie on the basis of money due in respect of work carried out, whether or not the money has been received, while at the same time money due in respect of expenses incurred can be claimed against tax, whether or not the practitioner has settled his bills for such expenses. In the event that the practitioner is subsequently unable to recover money due for which he has already paid tax, he can ask for such 'bad debts' to be taken into account as an expense in a later tax assessment.

After the practitioner has been in practice privately for three years it is possible to ask the Inland Revenue to change the basis of assessment from an earnings basis to a cash or receipts basis, ie paying tax on money *actually* received and receiving an allowance for expenses *actually* incurred. The Inland Revenue will agree to such a change only if it is more likely to provide a reasonable indication of the taxpayer's profits. However, any doctor wishing to effect such a change will be required to give a written undertaking to issue bills for services rendered at regular and frequent intervals.

Period of assessment and timing of payments

The Inland Revenue will issue an estimate of liability for tax and national insurance at the end of the fiscal year. On receipt of the assessment the practitioner has 30 days in which to appeal against the assessment and to submit a claim to postpone any of the income tax and class 4 national insurance contributions payable. Very often an accountant will be able to negotiate a more favourable assessment by means of this appeal. Once the accounts have been agreed the Inland Revenue will issue a statement of liability showing payment due in two separate instalments on 1 January within and 1 July following the end of the tax year. Payments should be made promptly on the due date or the individual will be liable for interest due on the sums owing.

The practitioner's first set of accounts must be made up for a period of at least 12 months from the date he commences private practice, depending on the annual year end he has chosen. The practitioner can choose any date he wishes to be his accounting year end, provided he continues to apply that year end date consistently in subsequent accounting. The practitioner is advised to notify the Inland Revenue of the date he commences private practice and to make sure his tax affairs are in order at that time.

The current year's income tax liabilities are based on the previous year's profits and the fiscal year runs to 5 April. It is therefore customary to adopt 30 April as the year end date as this will delay the income tax liability on a particular year's profits for the longest time. For instance, the income tax on profits for the year ended 30 April 1991 would form the basis of assessment for 1992/93 and the income tax would be payable on 1 January 1993 and 1 July 1993 in two equal instalments. If the annual accounts had been made up to 31 March 1991 the income tax would, however, be payable a year earlier as the accounts would form the basis of assessment for 1991/92.

However, in the opening years of a business special rules apply whereby the first year's profits will form the basis of assessment for the subsequent three years. Even though profits in the second and third years may greatly exceed the opening year, the Inland Revenue cannot increase the assessment for those years. Once the three years has ended, liability will be assessed on the basis of profits made during the last complete accounting year.

The date at which a practitioner ceases practice is also critical to the extent that the Revenue has the option to tax the consultant on his actual profits (instead of the preceding year's profits) for a period between two and three years before cessation, depending on the date when the practice is discontinued.

The assessment rules for partnership are similar to those for a doctor practising on his own although profits are divided between the partners for tax purposes on the basis of their profit-sharing ratios during the year of assessment. However, when a partner joins or leaves a practice, the Revenue will be obliged to regard the business of the partnership as having ended unless all the partners agree to be taxed on the normal preceding-year basis. Practice agreements should contain a clause requiring any retiring partner to sign a tax election as required by the remaining partners (to be signed as soon as possible after a new partner has joined the practice).

National Insurance

National Insurance liability adheres strictly to the tax classification. Consultants employed by the NHS will be paying the maximum national insurance contribution under class 1. They will not therefore be liable to pay class 2, the standard self-employed contribution (which is £5.55 per week in 1993/94) or class 4 contributions (an additional amount payable if practice profits exceed a certain limit subject to a maximum of £976.50 per annum during 1993/94.) To avoid overpayments and refunds after the year ends there is provision to apply for deferment of class 2 and class 4 contributions.

GPs and doctors wholly engaged in private practice will normally be liable for both class 2 and class 4 contributions. Class 2 contributions comprise a standard amount which is best paid four monthly by direct debit. Class 4 contributions are based on a percentage of profit above a certain limit which is assessed and becomes payable at the same time as income tax liability.

VAT

The supply of professional services by a registered medical practitioner and the supply of drugs and appliances by him in the course of his professional activities are exempt for VAT purposes. Medical practitioners do not therefore need to register for VAT or charge it to patients even where the practice turnover may exceed the registration limit (£36 000 in 1992/93). This means that the practitioner will be unable to recover VAT charged to him on items of expenditure connected with the practice and such expenses are not allowable against income tax.

Some practitioners have recently sought to register for VAT for the limited purpose of charging VAT in relation to equipment purchased or drugs dispensed on which they have incurred VAT liability. The merits and demerits of registering for VAT are too complex to be addressed here. In most cases registration will bring few benefits and practices should only consider doing so if their accountant believes strongly that there are genuine and permanent benefits to be derived from doing so.

Tax position of overseas doctors

UK tax liability is determined by the connection between the practitioner and the United Kingdom, ie whether he is regarded as resident, ordinarily resident or domiciled in this country.

A person may have only one place of domicile at any given time, and this denotes the country or state considered their permanent home regardless of residence or nationality. Being resident relates to their physical presence in the UK during a particular period. A person is ordinarily resident when they are 'habitually' so resident. The rules by which residence is determined are complex. However the basic test is whether the individual has been present in the UK for a period or periods which aggregate to 183 days or more during any one year, or 90 days or more a year over four years.

In general the UK resident is liable to UK income tax on UK and foreign income, whereas a non-resident is liable to UK income tax only on income earned in the UK. UK residents who are not domiciled in the UK or are Commonwealth or Irish citizens not ordinarily resident in the UK are generally assessed on foreign income remitted to the UK. Those coming to the UK to take up permanent residence are regarded as resident and ordinarily resident in the UK from the date of arrival.

References and further reading

British Medical Association (1993) *Tax Leaflet Series 1–6*. (Guidance notes).

British United Provident Association (1992) *A Guide to Private Consultant Practice*. BUPA London.

Elliot G K (1992) *'Start as You Mean to Go On': The Consultant's Practical and Financial Guide to Private Practice*. G.K. Elliot, Cheryls Close, London.

15

Pensions, Insurance and Finance

Superannuation

Where remuneration from private practice represents a substantial part of a doctor's income he would be well advised to set aside part of it in provision for his retirement. Doctors who devote the substantial part of their working life to the NHS will probably be members of the NHS pension scheme (NHSPS). As occupational pension schemes go, the NHSPS is highly regarded. In addition to a pension and lump sum payable at retirement the scheme offers significant ancillary benefits. Nevertheless the doctor engaging in private practice may need to supplement the benefits he will receive from it to avoid a significant shortfall in income upon his retirement.

To understand what considerations need to be borne in mind it will first be necessary to outline what the NHSPS involves.

NHS pension scheme

All NHS employed doctors, including whole-time salaried or part-time salaried consultants together with NHS GPs (although technically self-employed), are eligible for membership of the NHSPS. Prior to 6 April 1988 membership of the scheme was compulsory. It is now voluntary, but membership is automatic unless the doctor elects to opt out of the scheme.

Contributions to the NHSPS are paid from 'superannuable' earnings on the basis of a 4% contribution by the NHS and 6% by the doctor. Contributors are allowed full income tax relief on their contributions. GPs' superannuable pay relates only to remuneration in respect of NHS work and does not include the practice expenses deducted by the FHSA. The level of these expenses is determined each year by the Doctors and Dentists Review Body.

Consultants' superannuable earnings relate purely to their salaried employment in the NHS. Earnings of doctors generated from sources other than work under NHS contracts, such as private practice, lectures, research, writing books etc, do not qualify and are therefore classed as non-superannuable.

These earnings are normally assessable under Schedule D for tax purposes and can, therefore, be used for personal pension plan provision. Contributions to the NHS scheme are usually paid until the individual completes 45 years of service, or reaches age 70, or retires, if sooner.

On achieving 40 years service the doctor will be entitled to a pension at half the rate of final salary (usually the best of the last three years' superannuable remuneration) plus a single lump-sum payment at the rate of three times the pension. Anyone with 40 years service at age 60 can go on working in the NHS and get up to 45 years service for pension benefits. As an exception to the general rule any doctor working in psychiatry should be aware of the special provisions for mental health officers (who are able to retire at age 55).

Doctors are not permitted to contribute for more than 45 years of service in total to the NHSPS of which not more than 40 can accrue by age 60. However since most doctors qualify at about age 24 it is impossible for them to achieve, with normal working, their permitted maximum. Fortunately there are methods by which it is possible to cover at least some of any shortfall—the first is by purchasing added years.

Added years

This facility allows doctors to make tax-deductible additional payments to the NHSPS to bring their total superannuable service up to, or near the maximum allowed by age 60 (ie 40 years). The cost of each added year is a percentage of superannuable earnings which is determined by age at entry and repayment scale selected. The optimum extra contribution is 9% of salary, provided this does not acquire more than the maximum allowable number of Added Years. For example, under the scale where payments terminate at age 60, any doctor under 50 can purchase four added years for less than the stipulated 9%.

Purchase of Added Years increases pension, lump-sum and all ancillary benefits of the NHSPS. Contributions must continue until the end of the selected term unless ill health or financial hardship intervene.

The second means of covering any shortfall is by means of additional voluntary contributions.

Additional voluntary contributions

Since October 1987, doctors in occupational pension schemes have also been able to contribute to 'free-standing additional voluntary contribution schemes' (FSAVCS) in order to make up their pension. FSAVCS can be used to increase the pension only, not the lump sum. Doctors (with the exception of GPs) may pay FSAVCS in respect of all taxable income, not only on that which is superannuable under the occupational pension scheme. They will, therefore, be allowed on certain extra non-superannuable earnings, such as payments to junior doctors for additional duty hours or to other doctors for additional sessions. The Inland Revenue specifies that the total benefits at retirement age must not exceed two thirds of final remuneration. Any surplus from FSAVCS must be refunded at a special taxation rate.

There are several significant differences between FSAVCS and added years.

1   They provide only additional pension and no tax free cash. They do not enhance automatically the ancillary benefits of the NHSPS.

2   What they produce depends upon two variables not present in the NHSPS:
    — the performance of the fund into which contributions are invested
    — the annuity rates ruling when that fund must be converted from cash into pension.
    (Either or both of these could be beneficial or detrimental to the contributor.)

3   Unlike added years, payments to an FSAVCS may be changed by the doctor. Provided they are always within the limits defined by the Revenue, contributions may be increased, decreased, terminated or suspended, and reinstated. Thus they provide greater flexibility in this context than added years.

4   For doctors whose age at entry means that the 9% tax-deductible contribution limit cannot purchase the full entitlement of added years, the FSAVCS can provide more retirement income subject to the two variables detailed in 2 above.

5   GPs who, with normal working, will accrue more than 38.1 years of superannuable service by age 60, are presently precluded from contributing to an FSAVCS.

6   These schemes are available from many life assurance companies and other pension providers.

'In-house' AVC Scheme

In 1991 the NHSPS introduced a facility, which they arranged with the Equitable Life Assurance Society, by which members of the NHSPS could take out a contract to pay for in-scheme money to purchase additional voluntary contributions in order to increase their own pensions, increase their dependants' pension or increase the lump-sum paid on death.

The publicity for this scheme suggests that its administrative costs are minimal. With one exception, this 'in-house' facility is similar to FSAVCS. The essential difference is that doctors in general practice can purchase extra service under this scheme so their total does not exceed 40 years by age 60. In other words, unlike FSAVCS, practitioners are not restricted by the 38.1 years limit (*see* 5 in previous section).

The advantage of using the AVC arrangements offered by the NHSPS is that administrative costs are minimal. All contributions made in this regard will be deducted from income and attract tax relief. The maximum contribution which can be made towards AVCs is 9% of superannuable pay, depending on age and length of service. Contributions can be made annually, monthly or weekly and the amount paid can be varied or stopped at any time. The contributions will be invested by Equitable Life, or any other company chosen, in the way the doctor prefers with either profits investment, unit linked investment or via a deposit account. It will be possible for doctors to contribute to both added years and an FSAVCS.

The FSAVCS are obviously a more flexible method of contributing for extra pension. Contributions may be varied at any time whereas Added Years require a commitment of a fixed percentage of superannuable pay to be made right up to the chosen age of retirement. Contributions to an FSAVCS are made net of basic rate tax and higher rate tax can be reclaimed by an adjustment to the tax coding. It is important, however, that benefits accruing under FSAVCS are monitored regularly to prevent overfunding.

Added years, on the other hand, have to be paid gross and all the tax relief has to be reclaimed by adjustment to the assessments. However, added years can purchase an extra lump-sum on pension benefits whereas a FSAVCS only provides for additional pension benefits. Clearly there are merits and demerits of both FSAVC and added years. Individuals would therefore be well advised to seek independent financial advice on the benefits to be derived from each.

Personal pensions

A personal pension plan is a highly tax-efficient means of providing for retirement. It can be used to secure a pension for life, plus a tax-free lump-sum. There are four possible applications for doctors:

An alternative to the NHSPS

Since benefits from personal pensions may be taken at any time from age 50 (but must commence by age 75) they can provide retirement benefits earlier than those available under the NHSPS. With the latter the earliest date for payment of normal retirement benefits is age 60 unless the retirement is on grounds of ill-health.

Where a personal pension is in lieu of NHSPS there is no 4% contribution from the NHS. Furthermore these contracts do not include all the ancillary benefits that form an integral part of the NHSPS. Unlike the NHSPS personal pensions depend upon the two variables already mentioned, namely fund performance and annuity rates, to achieve their results.

However there are no 'emerging benefit' restrictions so, in theory, a personal pension could provide greater retirement benefits (pension and lump-sum) than is possible with the NHSPS. On the other hand, such benefits could equally well be inferior to those emanating from the NHSPS.

Whilst there is no universal formula for all doctors, it is likely that the majority will derive the most satisfactory results by accruing basic retirement benefits under the NHSPS for NHS earnings when all benefits from the scheme are taken into consideration, and use a personal plan for non-NHS earnings only.

Any doctor wishing to leave the NHSPS and make future provision for NHS earnings with personal pensions may only transfer to the latter NHS benefits that have been acquired since April 1988. Transfer of earlier accrued benefits is permitted only where the doctor no longer works in the NHS.

For earnings from non-NHS sources

As already mentioned, unless personal pension provision is made for such earnings nothing will replace them when they terminate. Meanwhile, attractive tax savings and efficient investment opportunities will have been lost.

For non-superannuable NHS earnings

If taxable earnings from the NHS for a GP exceed superannuable remuneration the difference constitutes 'net relevant earnings' for which private pension provision is permitted. In addition, the previous paragraph has equal relevance for such GPs.

Foregoing tax relief on contributions to the NHSPS

Since the tax relief available to GPs on contributions to the NHSPS is concessionary rather than statutory it need not be claimed. In such circumstances the Revenue allow personal pension provision to be made in respect of earnings already superannuated under the NHSPS. This double provision has been possible for many years and is a useful means of enhancing, significantly, income in retirement. However it involves a substantial increase in net expenditure and any practitioner pursuing this path should ensure that a proper comparison is made of both cost and benefits 'before and after'. A particular attraction of this facility is that a decision whether or not to claim tax relief on NHSPS contributions may be taken annually. Thus a continuing commitment is not necessary.

Contributions

Payments to personal pensions, which attract full tax relief, are subject to maxima which depend upon age. The maximum contribution levels are as follows:

Age ≤ 35 — 17.5% of net relevant earnings

Age 36–45 years — 20% of net relevant earnings

Age 46–50 years — 25% of net relevant earnings

Age 51–55 years — 30% of net relevant earnings

Age 56–60 years — 35% of net relevant earnings

Age ≥ 61 years years — 40% of net relevant earnings.

Important disadvantages of personal pensions are that, unlike the NHS pension scheme, the final benefits are not necessarily index-linked, and additional special insurance will have to be taken out to safeguard against ill-health etc.

It is possible and can be in the doctor's interest to elect to forego the tax relief available to the NHSPS and to redirect the tax relief to contributions in a personal pension plan. This means the doctor can maximize benefits taken from a personal pension plan and still enjoy the benefits from the NHSPS. It is a unique privilege allowed by the Inland Revenue only to members of the NHS pension scheme.

Obviously the type of personal plan chosen and the benefits offered will vary enormously. Again, independent financial advice is essential in order to determine the most suitable for the individual concerned.

Life assurance considerations

If a member of the NHSPS with more than two years' service dies in service, their widow (or widower, provided certain extra requirements have been complied with) will receive an initial pension. This will be equivalent to the deceased's superannuable pay for between three and six months. Thereafter it will equate to the pension that would have been payable had the deceased retired on grounds of ill-health on the day he or she died. Additional allowances are payable in respect of dependent children.

There are several ways of calculating the death gratuity, but the two methods most likely to be applicable are either (1) one year's final superannuable pay or (2) the lump-sum payable had the member retired on the grounds of ill-health on the day before death. The first method is more likely to be applicable if death occurs in the years leading up to retirement but, clearly, if death occurs soon after joining the NHS, the second method will be better. However, it is unlikely that the amount allowable in the death gratuity and death benefit allowances will be sufficient to meet the needs of a practitioner's dependents after his death. It is therefore advisable to take out additional protection in the form of life assurance policies.

The cheapest form of cover is term assurance. This provides a tax-free lump-sum and/or income if death occurs during a period determined when the policy is completed. Nothing is payable if the practitioner survives the selected term, which is the reason why such cover is inexpensive. However, he may be able to receive tax relief on the premium if it is made solely from private practice income. No more than 5% of such income may be made for this purpose.

Many forms of life assurance policy are available beyond simple term assurance, most of which involve an element of investment bringing with them the possibility of a financial return of some kind at maturity. The number of policies available is enormous and have many features which may affect initial costs, ongoing costs and benefits ultimately payable. To ensure the best deal possible in the circumstances, practitioners are again advised to seek independent financial advice.

Sickness and personal medical insurance

Any member of the NHSPS who has completed two or more years' service and is unable through permanent ill-health or other disability to continue in their present form of work can apply for an ill-health pension. This is payable without prejudice to the contributor's ability to do a different type of work. All NHS doctors, including GPs, are covered under the NHS injury benefits scheme whilst engaged on NHS duties. This is non-contributory and separate from the NHS pension scheme. However, in the event that these benefits do not offer sufficient income to the practitioner affected, it may be advisable to take out protection against loss of income due to illness or incapacity by establishing a permanent health insurance plan, and possibly a critical illness plan.

A permanent health insurance plan will pay out a regular income if the practitioner falls ill or has an accident which results in either a temporary or permanent cessation of earnings. A critical illness plan provides a cash lump-sum following the diagnosis of such illnesses as heart attack, cancer, stroke, kidney failure, paralysis or some other form of permanent disablement before the age of 60, or the necessity for bypass surgery or major organ transplant. These policies can sometimes be linked to investments so the advice of an independent financial advisor should be sought about such matters. Any income payable from such policies is normally free of tax until the benefit has been paid for a complete fiscal year. However premiums payable are not tax deductible, though tax relief is available for the over 60s on personal medical insurance (*see* below).

The multiplicity and complexity of these policies make independent financial advice essential when such cover is being considered. It should be noted that receipt by a practitioner of an ill-health retirement pension under the NHSPS does not preclude the recipient from working in the NHS subsequently. It may be possible to retain pension and work in the NHS where the work is qualitatively different or of sufficiently reduced capacity.

In the event that the privately practising doctor requires private treatment himself, it obviously makes sense to have some form of private medical insurance. This will ensure that the period of incapacity covered by the illness and its treatment are kept to a minimum. It is of course an old tradition in the medical profession that doctors should not charge colleagues or their dependents for treatment (*see* Chapter 8). It is on the basis of this tradition that discounts are offered to members of the special health insurance schemes offered to members of the BMA by BUPA and PPP. Some other health insurance schemes are now being established which are apparently tailored to the needs of the medical profession. However there has been a suggestion that benefits offered by the latter do not compare favourably with schemes available to the public because doctors are considered to be a high risk as far as health insurance is concerned! Presumably this is based on a perception that doctors, being familiar with the need for treatment and the availability of it, are more likely to make use of their health insurance policies than members of the public. Whatever the truth of such perceptions, it is advisable to study a number of alternatives available before making up one's mind about the health insurance scheme to adopt.

Both BMA schemes comprise two alternative schemes, one being cheaper and less comprehensive than the other. These schemes, and others available to doctors, involve contributions based to a certain degree on claims made within certain age bandings. As a result, subscriptions tend to escalate the older one gets in recognition of the fact that the risk of ill-health increases proportionately. There is not normally any no claims bonus or equivalent available within such schemes.

Other insurance considerations

A private practitioner employing staff will need to take out employers' liability insurance to provide cover for legal liability for injuries to employees in his service attributed to his negligence. In addition he should obtain separate cover for legal liability for injuries to 'visitors' to the premises arising from negligence by him or any of his employees. Contents and equipment insurance is another essential, particularly where expensive equipment is vital to the practice; it may also be advisable to consider additional forms of insurance such as that which provides cover against the cost of professional fees incurred as a result of such contingencies as disputes with landlords, Inland Revenue investigations, and problems surrounding the supply of goods and services. Many insurance companies now offer composite schemes which provide cover for the majority of a practitioner's insurance requirements.

Financial assistance

When setting up in private practice for the first time, the practitioner may well have to borrow a substantial sum, either to secure the lease of premises he requires or to purchase equipment necessary for him to practise privately. Fortunately most financial institutions regard doctors as a 'good bet' financially speaking, though they are more likely to be favourably inclined towards a doctor in NHS practice who is merely seeking to supplement his income from private sources. Most high-street banks will be prepared to offer loans on reasonable terms but there are a number of financial institutions who are prepared to offer special financial deals for doctors.

For the really substantial financial outlay required in purchasing freehold premises or having them built, as GPs commonly do, a special financial institution set up by the government, but acquired a few years ago by Norwich Union, known as the General Practice Finance Corporation (GPFC), is an avenue worth considering. Whilst their area of interest is principally that of general practice, with particular emphasis on cost rent schemes, they are not adverse to lending money to doctors for other purposes, and count some private practitioners among their clientele.

The address of the GPFC is given in the Appendix. For financial guidance in a wider context, two companies are pre-eminent: BMA Services Ltd (BMAS), a company part-owned by the BMA, which specializes in advising doctors on the best insurance and financial deals available and is able to offer a range of discounts and benefits to BMA members; and the Medical Insurance Agency (MIA), a company with a long history of service to the medical profession, which is unusual in donating one third of its profits to healthcare charities. Addresses for both companies may be found at the back of the book.

References and further reading

British Medical Association (1993) *Superannuation: A Guide For Medical Practitioners*. (Guidance note).

16

Some Specialist Considerations

Throughout this book we have referred to the situation of specialists as an undifferentiated group. In this chapter we will seek to consider some problems which affect individual, mainly non-surgical, specialties.

Anaesthetics

As we have seen, the group practice or combine is becoming an increasingly common feature among anaesthetists. One reason for this is the high cost of equipment required.

Equipment

Anaesthetists practising individually may yet have at least some of their own equipment. This may be purchased second-hand from other anaesthetists, either via word of mouth or advertisements in professional journals. However it is usually advisable to have such equipment checked and if necessary overhauled by its manufacturers. When purchasing such equipment the anaesthetist must bear in mind the manufacturers' planned obsolescence of the equipment, and the future availability of spare parts and servicing facilities. Medical gas cylinders can, however, be hired easily and cheaply.

Drugs

NHS hospitals and most private hospitals will usually provide the full range of anaesthetic drugs for which they will make the appropriate charges. For those cases where the anaesthetist will be required to supply the drugs himself he will be wise to establish a relationship with his preferred neighbourhood pharmacist or pharmaceutical wholesaler. By buying locally it will be possible to save on the capital value of drugs kept in store, to ensure fresh supplies can be obtained speedily and efficiently and probably obtain a professional discount. Advice should be sought on the storage of drugs as appropriate from the BMA or defence organizations.

Dental anaesthetics

A considerable amount of private work is available to anaesthetists with respect to dental anaesthesia. About 400,000 dental operations involving general anaesthesia occur each year in the NHS alone. The system of payment for dental anaesthetics under the NHS is archaic and hopelessly inadequate for the needs of a proficient and well equipped service, as identified in the government report on the service produced by the working party chaired by Professor Poswillo. Unfortunately the system is founded on item of service fees payable to the dentist, whose level is calculated by the Doctors and Dentists Review Body as part of the dental profession's global remuneration for general dental services. Accordingly the rate, which has always been niggardly and inappropriate, was actually reduced in April 1991 following the well publicized clawback of general dental practitioners' remuneration authorized by the government as a consequence of an alleged over-payment during 1990/91.

Proposals for a radical overhaul of the system are now being considered. In the meantime it is clear that anaesthetists will increasingly have little interest in such work, other than as a means of establishing a professional relationship with local dentists through whom they may expect to inherit a volume of private cases.

The exodus of general dental practitioners from the NHS as a consequence of their dispute with the government over pay during 1991/92 has undoubtedly increased the number of dental cases requiring general anaesthesia being undertaken privately. In any event it is common for dental practitioners to provide the equipment used by the anaesthetist. However the requirements recommended by the Poswillo Report will undoubtedly limit the provision of dental anaesthesia to a small number of large general dental group practices or specialist dental practices to which other dentists will refer patients requiring general anaesthesia. It is difficult to see how else the high standards can be maintained for dental anaesthetics outside the NHS or private hospitals.

During 1992/93 the Government made £9 million available in grants to enable general dental practitioners and 'others involved in the provision of general anaesthesia services in dentistry' to uprate their equipment to the recommended standards. The means by which this money was distributed via regional health authorities varied from region to region. It is doubtful whether very much of it was taken up by anaesthetists, however, and it is not known whether further grants are to be made available in future.

Reimbursement of anaesthetists' fees

As we have noted, health insurers formerly lumped together anaesthetists' fees with those payable to surgeons in calculations of benefits reimbursed for subscribers' treatment. Often the surgeon received the whole amount and passed on a previously agreed percentage to the anaesthetist whom he had engaged to provide the anaesthetic. It was generally assumed that the anaesthetist should receive approximately one third of the total fee. The Association of Anaesthetists objected to the existence of this differential, noting (with some justification) that the contribution made by anaesthetists varied depending on the operation, so that on some occasions the amount properly due as a reflection of the skill and degree of responsibility owned by the anaesthetist could be much higher than one third. The Association published its own scale of fees for anaesthetics, which enjoyed considerable currency. However it was obviously essential from their point of view to have the agreement of the major health insurers. A series of heated discussions between the Association and BUPA resulted in a compromise following a major shift in position on the part of the insurers.

In the meantime the BMA guidelines had contributed to the breakdown of the old 2:1 ratio in fees by publishing a separate scale of fees for anaesthetists which were not directly related to the work of the surgeon. In 1992, following months of negotiations with the Association of Anaesthetists, BUPA decided to follow suit. It could only do so, however, by virtue of a substantial extra cash injection to boost anaesthetists' fees above the one third level where required without corresponding reductions in surgeons' fees.

The second largest insurer, PPP, has so far resisted the move towards separate anaesthetists' fees. Each operation in its schedule of procedures is given a single banding in terms of degree of difficulty covering both surgeon and anaesthetist. One particular problem which arises from this which is that where reimbursement is limited to a particular amount, as is the case with PPP plans involving hospital bands B, C and D, for instance, surgeons and anaesthetists may find themselves in competition with each other in obtaining the share of reimbursement they consider due. Because PPP reimburse on a 'first-come first-served' basis, it is possible for the first consultant to receive full reimbursement of his bill, leaving a correspondingly smaller amount for the second consultant. In practice it is usually the surgeon who suffers most as the result of this arrangement, as anaesthetists, particularly those in anaesthetic combines, are recognized as being more punctilious in submitting bills for their services. PPP has so far shown no willingness to amend its procedures in recognition of such difficulties.

Obstetrics and 'fertility regulation'

Demand for private obstetrics

Obstetrics is, as we have already noted, unusual among acute specialists in that demand for private specialist services is unrelated to waiting-lists. There are, by definition, no waiting-lists in obstetrics though there may well be in the related specialty of gynaecology. The reasons why patients opt to go private when giving birth must therefore relate in large part to a desire for comfort and privacy, more attentive nursing and the personal service of the obstetrician. For many, anxieties about giving birth will be allayed by knowing that a senior obstetrician will be on hand to deal with their confinement, and the discomfort and stress of labour will be alleviated by the more comfortable and less pressurized surroundings of a private labour suite.

Limits of health insurance

Obstetrics is also unusual in that it is not provided for by health insurance. The reasons for this lie in the rationale for health insurance. This is stated in most policies to be to provide for the 'cure or relief' of 'acute illness or injury'. Pregnancy is not an illness or injury and is unique among medical conditions in being, in most cases, voluntarily incurred. Health insurance is based on assessment of risk factors associated with involuntary processes and it would generally be considered unwise, in insurance terms, to provide cover for someone who may choose to incur this expense with an unknown degree of frequency.

Of course health insurance policies do sometimes provide cover for relief of acute illness and injury which arise from and during pregnancy, including, in some cases, therapeutic abortions. The list of procedures, however, as will be seen from the most recent BUPA schedule, remains very limited. Almost all private obstetrics will be paid for by patients. While private labour suites are a mainstay of many private hospitals, occupancy of pay beds in NHS hospitals by patients treated by obstetricians is relatively high. It has also proved to be an area where NHS Trusts are pioneering the availability of hotel services to private patients.

Abortion and fertility services

Obstetricians and gynaecologists may also expect to be able to undertake a significant amount of private practice in 'fertility regulation'. This is the term used to cover termination of pregnancy, sterilization and treatment of fertility problems, almost none of which are covered by health insurance. Abortion is an area of medical care where the NHS has never provided a fully comprehensive service. The gaps in the service have largely been filled by charitable, and to a lesser extent commercial, abortion clinics. A total of 180 000 abortions were carried out in England and Wales in 1991, of which 104 000 were in the independent sector. Most of the commercial clinics' clientele come from outside the UK.

High-technology treatments for infertility such as in vitro fertilization have largely been developed in the private sector. While their availability in the NHS remains controversial and a victim of the present debate on rationing of services, such treatments look set to remain an area in which the private sector will continue to remain dominant.

Pathology

Pathology is a specialty which it is difficult to equate with the usual perception of private practice and the definition of it in the NHS Terms and Conditions of Service. In every other specialty, private practice usually involves direct contact with patients. Pathology involves specimens taken from patients.

Private laboratories

There are a number of wholly private laboratories staffed by consultant pathologists who are also employed by the NHS. A number of private hospitals also have their own pathology services, often supervised on a part-time basis by NHS-employed consultants. A common situation is for the pathologist to contract with the private hospital to provide a consultant service in return for a retaining fee, often with some additional remuneration on an item-of-service basis. Consultants thinking of entering into such an arrangement should establish how many patients will be involved, in order to decide whether to relinquish their whole-time contract in favour of a maximum part-time contract. Setting individual fees and retainers so low that earnings from private practice do not exceed the 10% limit may be unwise and lead to problems should the amount of private work increase.

It is considered advisable for the pathologist to involve himself fully in the running of any private laboratory with which he is concerned, exactly as he would in his NHS department, rather than adopt a purely visiting role. The pathologist will also need to establish whether he is expected to provide a locum during periods of absence.

Laing (1993) recorded 138 private pathology laboratories operating in the UK, and also 30 exclusively in-house laboratories sited in private hospitals having no need to sell services to third parties. Only a very small number of these describe themselves as research, reference or forensic laboratories. Between 1989 and 1991 competition among private laboratories increased with the arrival of a number of new companies attracted by the prospect of NHS privatization. However, as the 1991 annual report of one of the largest organizations, J S Pathology, noted, 'minimal opportunities have been found so far for working with the NHS'.

Since then private pathology laboratories have faced increased competition from health authorities keen to generate revenue by selling pathology services. However there are undoubtedly increased opportunities for joint collaboration ventures. A number of on-site private hospital laboratories are already run under contract and there is no reason why private pathology companies should not manage NHS laboratories or run them on behalf of health authorities as commercial ventures.

Private pathology fees in NHS hospitals

When working in NHS hospitals the consultant treating the private patient is supposed to arrange for the processing of specimens taken from the patient privately. Having informed the patient that an additional charge will be levied for this service, he is supposed to ensure that the appropriate fee is passed on to his pathologist colleagues. The 'primary' consultant has this responsibility because, as the pathologist will never see the patient, he will have no way of knowing whether the specimens came from a private patient, unless the primary consultant has so designated the specimen. If private work is sent to an NHS laboratory, the pathologist in charge must make sure that any payment due to the NHS authority concerned from the patient is forthcoming.

Pathologists are often asked to process specimens from deceased patients (eg for post-mortem examinations), or non-human agents such as river water samples, on a private basis. In these circumstances there is often considerable debate as to whether such work is category 2 or some other kind of private work which does not fall within the definition of category 2 but which cannot be regarded as private practice either. The unique nature of pathology causes many such problems.

Collection of private fees

The principal difficulty with private pathology in the NHS is the fact that the volume of work carried out and the small cost of the individual items processed militates against submission of proper invoices. This has led to a situation whereby pathologists frequently allow the NHS hospital to collect their fees and rely on the hospital to pass on the income derived to them after deduction of an appropriate fee for administration. This is all very well in theory, but in practice there are a number of attendant problems. Unless the pathologist keeps a careful check of the specimens he has processed it is very difficult to know whether the hospital has, by accident or design, not paid the pathologist all the monies he is due. Arrangements for collection of pathology fees vary from one hospital to another, as do the administrative charges.

Any pathologist taking up a consultant post for the first time is advised to obtain precise information about the cost of such charges. He will also need to be sure to separate out the fees in respect of private patients which will contribute towards his 10% limit, those which are exempt from any charge, eg coroners' post-mortem examinations, and those which are accepted as being category 2 work of which one third is due in payment to the hospital, eg coroners' analytical work.

In some cases pathologists may find themselves paying an administrative fee composed of a percentage, eg 10% to 20% of each fee collected, while still having to remit one third of some of their fees to the hospital. The newly appointed pathologist should be wary of this situation but may find that he is hidebound by local custom and practice.

Post-mortem examinations

The status of coroners' post-mortem examinations is something of a historical anomaly. The reason why pathologists do not have to remit one third of these fees to their employing authority is principally because in most places in the UK the hospital mortuary doubles as the public mortuary and as such is partially funded by the local authority. Because of this contribution (whether real or merely hypothetical), the NHS hospital is precluded from demanding one third of the pathologist's fee. This does not apply to other analytical work for the coroner of which one third of the fee is payable. The status of the purely private post-mortem examination, that is where the relatives of the deceased wish to pay for a second opinion, is not altogether clear. It certainly does not accord with the definition of private practice, but as it is invariably carried out in the public mortuary by an independent pathologist, category 2 fees are not necessarily appropriate either. Though commonly regarded as private practice, this remains something of a grey area.

Provision of NHS services to third parties

Pathology services are something which many NHS hospitals, especially Trusts, are keen to sell to third parties like private hospitals on a block contract basis. Sometimes this will provide additional remuneration to the pathologist concerned and sometimes not. Many pathologists have rightly queried whether their employing hospital has the right to provide pathology services to third parties without the consent of the consultants involved. Where the pathologists work under contracts still governed by the national Terms and Conditions of Service, paragraph 31 of the same dictates that the hospital cannot so contract with a third party without the agreement of the practitioner concerned. This paragraph provides that the pathologists may in that situation negotiate directly, with the third party concerned, appropriate fees for the services in question. Alternatively they may reach agreement with their employing authority to be paid for this work by means of additional NHS sessions.

Of course the position of NHS Trusts puts a completely different complexion on such arrangements. Under locally negotiated contracts, pathologists may find their ability to receive separate remuneration for non-NHS work extremely circumscribed. Even work involving coroners' post-mortem examinations may be affected. Some Trusts are believed to have negotiated arrangements with their pathologists whereby all coroners' post-mortem examinations are undertaken as part of normal contractual duties, for which the pathologist will receive no additional remuneration, the coroners' fees being paid directly to the Trust.

Indeed the nature of pathology, in having no direct contact with private patients, means that it is relatively easy for employing authorities to sidestep the time-honoured practices referred to in the Green Book. The pathologists' employers may argue, with some justification, that 'a specimen is a specimen' and that there are no 'personal services' which the pathologist can render to the patient in these circumstances which would differentiate NHS from private work. Pathology is likely, therefore, to be one area in which NHS Trusts may seek to exclude all opportunities for consultants to benefit from private practice, and experience so far suggests that there will be little that can be done to halt this development.

Taxation of fees

The provision of pathology services to third parties (known formally as Section 58 services) is commonplace and can be quite a money spinner for the hospital. In university medical establishments many pathologists have traditionally not had the ability to keep fees derived from private work, these being paid into academic or educational trust funds used to purchase equipment for the department or pay for educational courses. However this has led on occasion to difficulties with the Inland Revenue. It is essential for the individuals concerned to ascertain whether the Revenue accepts such funds as having 'charitable status' or else the pathologists may find themselves having a resultant tax liability for the private fees earned.

Pathologists should be careful also about payments made to NHS hospital staff assisting them as this can create problems for those staff vis-à-vis their employers and the Inland Revenue, and may cause the pathologist tax problems. It is therefore quite common for pathologists to pay monies for the services of NHS staff assisting them, usually about 10% of fees received, into departmental funds for equipment. Monies paid for in this way are fully tax-deductible.

Psychiatry

Private clinics

As we have already noted, private psychiatric treatment is potentially very costly. The majority of psychiatric patients who need to get away from home require treatment in a positively therapeutic environment. Because of the expense this involves, specialist intermural psychiatric care was more often left to the NHS but recent moves towards care in the community, coupled with the closure of many of the large State institutions, have paved the way for private psychiatric hospital development. The result is that acute psychiatric treatment has been one of the minor focal points of growth in the private sector in recent years.

There are at least two large groups of private psychiatric hospitals, the Priory Group and the Charter Clinics, as well as a number of smaller independent clinics and charitable institutions. The private clinics have tended to have a small number of full-time consultant staff and a larger number of visiting consultants who have NHS consultant appointments and who depend on fee income for their private earnings.

Recently both the Priory and Charter Groups have pioneered what is described as an 'open-staff' model in which local psychiatric consultants have admitting rights. The Priory Group has also developed a 'semi-open' or 'mixed-staff' model as its hospital in South-West London. The remaining non-NHS providers have also started to experiment with admitting rights for consultant psychiatrists not on the hospital staff.

Both in the NHS and the private sector the trend is now firmly in favour of extramural care, and the bulk of psychiatric care is on an out-patient basis. Fees are almost entirely based on consultations, as it is the consultation itself which is the principal mode of treatment. A study by Wilkinson in 1988 estimated that in 1986 there were 300 psychiatric consultants in Britain with a significant commitment to private practice, in addition to about 60 psychiatrists employed full-time in independent hospitals. Figures for both are likely to have increased since then in proportion to the increase in private places and the relative decline in NHS intramural provision.

Managed care

Unfortunately private medical insurance is geared towards in-patient treatment with only modest amounts allowed for consultations and out-patient treatment. A course of psychiatric treatment or psychotherapy may involve more than one consultation per week over a period of months or even years, so problems of reimbursement are not uncommon. Where in-patient treatment is allowed, the major insurers now operate managed care options involving either specific pre-authorization of admission or detailed reports on treatment carried out.

The difficulty for the health insurers as regards psychiatric treatment lies in properly determining when a course of treatment has been completed or indeed whether it has been successful. PPP has adopted a 'velvet glove' approach to managed care in psychiatric treatment (*see* Chapter 5). Full-blown managed care is seen as impractical in psychiatry because it is impossible to develop precise clinical protocols which will satisfy all schools of psychiatric thought. As part of this approach, PPP requires hospitals to provide them with:

- ICD diagnosis (or confirm admission to facilitate diagnosis)
- a verified treatment plan

- the expected date of discharge.

As from 1992 BUPA introduced an even more rigorous regime involving pre-authorization and utilization review following lengthy and constructive discussions with the Royal College of Psychiatrists. This comprised the following elements:

- No in-patient or day-patient costs for psychiatric/addictive illness are to be incurred without BUPA's prior knowledge and written agreement (subject to special arrangements for emergency admissions).

- Full medical reports and medical history are to be provided before BUPA will enter into written agreements to meet such costs.

- Benefits will not be payable for more than 90 days in a year for any given patient.

- The hospital must be a registered mental nursing-home.

- No benefits are payable for treatment arising from any chronic or recurrent mental or addictive condition or disorder.

- No benefits are payable for treatment for any mental or addictive condition or disorder if it is received within two years of joining BUPA.

Category 2 work

Psychiatrists employed by the NHS may find themselves being asked, and sometimes pressurized, into accepting a good deal of category 2 work. One major area of such work takes the form of collaborative arrangement services, eg assisting social services with reports, assessments and attendance at case conferences as necessary regarding patients needing psychiatric care in the community, or determining whether individuals are sufficiently well mentally to look after themselves or their children.

Psychiatrists may also be asked to undertake assessments for various legal purposes, eg in determining the degree of psychological trauma or 'nervous shock' to be attributed to an accident which is the subject of a compensation claim, or making an assessment of a person's ability to manage their own affairs in relation to an application for Power of Attorney or for the Court of Protection.

Legal work is often remunerative, especially for those who concentrate on appearing as expert witnesses in court, but it can be very time-consuming. Psychiatrists often complain of finding it impossible to undertake the work of preparing reports for legal proceedings other than in their own time. They also frequently complain about attempts by their employing health authorities to charge them for the use of their consulting rooms for the consultations with patients preliminary to the preparation of such reports. Once again it is a failure on the part of the hospital authorities properly to understand the distinction between category 2 and private practice which is at fault.

Communication with GPs

One difficulty faced by psychiatrists in private practice lies in the special interpretation of 'private' by certain patients who take it to mean, not as it should mean, private from the NHS, but 'private from the general practitioner'. It is often assumed to be acceptable to conceal psychiatric consultation from GPs when undertaken privately. The reason given is usually that the GP does not understand or is liable to be unsympathetic to such treatment or he is so intimate a family friend that it would be embarrassing for the material to be communicated. Psychiatrists should be extremely wary of bypassing their patient's general practitioner: first, because it undermines the principle of GPs being the gatekeeper or co-ordinator of secondary treatment; secondly, because it underlines the widely held but wrong-headed belief that psychiatry is outside ordinary medicine; and thirdly, because such bypassing makes prescribing appropriate medication impossible for fear that the GP, uninformed of its nature, might himself prescribe something incompatible with the psychiatrist's prescription.

Further problems evinced by psychiatrists are the domestic problem of private patients telephoning them at home often at any hour regarding any developments in preference to consulting their family doctor. Psychiatrists should be wary of seeing a patient in such circumstances without informing their GP. They should make it clear to patients that armed with this information, the GP is likely to be in the best position to deal with such matters in the interim between consultations.

It is often considered useful for a psychiatrist in private practice to have access to a psychologist who is both good at functional and/or organic psychiatric testing, particularly if the psychiatrist in private practice deals with medico-legal work, like compensation cases.

Ethics of private psychiatry

The question of patient consent is a familiar problem but has recently been put under the spotlight by examples of disturbing cases in the USA reported in the UK press. These involved apparently sane patients, showing signs of anxiety or distress as a normal consequence of unfortunate developments in their private lives, being incarcerated in private mental institutions against their will, apparently for no other reason than the profit to be derived from their treatment via health insurance. A documentary television programme reported that the company responsible was intent on establishing private psychiatric clinics in the UK. All right-thinking psychiatrists will be justly horrified at the suggestion that such cases might find a parallel in this country. Fortunately the limited amount of reimbursement available via health insurance, the small numbers of potential claimants, and the regime of managed care instituted by the major health insurers will militate against such developments. It has nevertheless served to give private psychiatrists pause for thought.

Radiology

Many of the comments made above in relation to anaesthesia and pathology apply to radiology but for the radiologist one benefit of private practice is the ability to offer a more personal service to the patient than he is at liberty to do in his NHS environment. He may feel he is able to play a greater part in the treatment of the patient by being on hand to give the patient and the referring specialist the benefit of his opinion on the case in a more direct manner.

Equipment

NHS or private hospital equipment can often be used but group practices are commonly the only means by which radiologists can themselves afford to provide the equipment necessary to exercise their skills to the full. While X-ray machines are not beyond the resources of individuals, the more sophisticated types of scanning equipment, eg for CT and MRI are obviously very expensive and rarely available outside hospitals. As has been noted, radiologists using private facilities must acquaint themselves with the requirement of the Ionizing Radiation Regulations (*see* Chapter 11) particularly as regards health and safety and the necessity of employing only appropriately qualified staff. In a group practice a radiographer can be employed to handle casual chest X-rays etc as well as assisting the radiologist and undertaking routine administrative work.

The problem of fees for the 'tertiary practitioner'

Radiologists face particular problems when taking X-rays in NHS hospitals of fundholders' patients seen privately by consultant colleagues. The fact that the patients are NHS patients from whom no undertaking to pay has been received prevents them from levying a charge on the patient, and the fact that the fundholder has a contract with the hospital prevents them levying an additional charge on the fundholder. Many, including the Private Practice and Professional Fees Committee of the BMA and the Joint Subcommittee of the Joint Consultants Committee and the Central Consultants and Specialists Committee of the BMA on Independent Medical Practice, consider that, in these circumstances, it behoves the fundholder and the 'secondary' practitioner to include in the contract between them provision for payment to any 'tertiary' practitioner who may be involved. Unfortunately there is no legal requirement to do this and it is to be doubted whether radiologists or pathologists can expect to receive any remuneration from such services.

Category 2 work

Radiologists can expect to undertake a reasonable amount of category 2 work, that is by way of providing radiological reports for insurers, solicitors, employers or government departments, eg in connection with sickness benefits, war pensions, accident/injury compensation claims etc. Where such work is undertaken at an NHS hospital the radiologist is obliged to pay one third of any fee received to his employing authority for the use of the technical equipment used. Non-routine screening of health authority employees also brings in category 2 fees.

In all these cases it is as well to remember the distinction between category 2 work (examples of which are listed in paragraph 37 of the Terms and Conditions of Service) and the definition of private practice in paragraph 40 of the same, namely the 'diagnosis or treatment of patients by private arrangement'. While the X-rays taken of the patient referred by an insurer for example, are undoubtedly diagnosis by private arrangement, there is clearly no element of treatment involved so that, as far as radiology is concerned, it may be thought that the definition should be regarded in practice as being more properly 'diagnosis arising from or which may reasonably be expected to be associated with, private treatment'. This is certainly how health authority lawyers are likely to regard the matter.

References and further reading

British United Provident Association (1992) *A Guide to Private Consultant Practice*. BUPA, London.

Central Committee for Hospital Medical Services, BMA (1984) *Pathology Services and Private Patients of Consultants: Suggested Code of Good Practice*. BMJ, London.

Central Committee for Hospital Medical Services, BMA (1985) *Radiology Services and Private Patients of Consultants: Suggested Code of Good Practice*. BMJ, London.

Department of Health and Social Security (1986) *A Guide to Private Practice in Health Service Hospitals in England and Wales*. DHSS, London.

Department of Health and Social Security (1984) *The Terms and Conditions of Service for Hospital Medical and Dental Staff*. DHSS, London.

J S Pathology (1991) *Report and Accounts for the year 1991*. JS Pathology, London.

Laing W (1993) *Laing's Review of Private Healthcare.* Laing & Buisson, London.

Poswillo DE (1990) *Report of the Standing Dental Advisory Committee on General Anaesthesia, Sedation and Resuscitation in Dentistry.* DoH, London.

Wilkinson G (1988) *Psychiatry: Private and Public Provision. British Medical Journal.* **296**:79.

17

Other Fee-paid Work

Scope of opportunities for private work

This book has been concerned with private practice defined in terms of treating private patients. But private practice can be seen in much broader terms, embracing various types of non-NHS fee-paid work available to doctors. For the sake of completeness this chapter aims to describe in broad outline some of the principal areas of such work, of which there is a bewildering variety involving sessional, hourly or item of service payments. BMA members may obtain further information on the subject from *Medical Careers: A General Guide* and from the guidance note *Fees for Part-Time Medical Services*, to which there are 35 individually available fees supplements, detailing fees and the circumstances in which they are paid in various areas: eg work for government departments, insurance medicals and reports, and medico-legal work. There are opportunities for all doctors to undertake such work but, due to the nature of their NHS contracts, it is once again consultants and GPs who are chiefly able to take advantage of these opportunities.

Medico-legal work

Medico-legal work can be one of the most lucrative areas of fee-paid work, but it is also one of the most complex and demanding. It would be pointless to try and describe the extraordinary complexities of the legal system in the UK (especially considering that it comprises two distinct legal systems), but fortunately there is a plethora of books available on the subject. The work for doctors arising from it consists mainly of reports based on examinations of patients or on records which are used for evidential purposes, and the giving of expert testimony in courts of law. For the consultant, medico-legal work is regarded as category 2 work (it is specifically referred to as such in paragraph 37 of the Terms and Conditions of Service). For GPs it is simply one of the many areas of private work (*see* Chapter 2).

There is an important distinction between work done in a *professional* capacity and work done in an *expert* capacity. The distinction is unrelated to experience or ability but refers to the status of the doctor vis-à-vis the subject of litigation or legal proceedings. If a doctor is asked to provide a factual report or give evidence in court on facts obtained from having acted in a professional capacity (for instance if he is asked to give a report about treatment given by him to a patient) he will be said to be acting as a professional witness. The rate of remuneration he will be offered will be consequently less than if he was an outsider, so to speak, specifically brought in by one of the parties to the proceedings to offer an opinion and interpret facts on the basis of his acknowledged expertise.

Nearly all doctors who deal with patients on a regular basis can expect to be asked to provide professional reports or testimony at some point in their careers. Almost all of these complain that payment for their services in such circumstances is inadequate. A smaller number of doctors are able to specialize in medico-legal work, offering their services as acknowledged experts in their particular specialties, and they are often able to command considerably more.

Unfortunately the amounts doctors are able to earn from such work, be they experts or acting in a professional capacity, are severely circumscribed whenever the cost of proceedings are funded by the public purse. In the majority of criminal cases the defence will be funded by Legal Aid so that both prosecution and defence are publicly funded. However in civil litigation also, although only one third of cases are funded by Legal Aid (and the number is diminishing), there are still restrictions on the amounts payable for reports and the services of professional witnesses, though less so for expert services. This is because the cost of medico-legal services which will normally fall upon the losing party is determined by the court (or a court official known as a taxing master) which may decide to allow less than the amount the doctor had originally asked for.

Consequently solicitors engaging doctors' services will rarely agree to payment before the case has been settled and only then agree to pay the doctor's 'reasonable' fees 'subject to taxation'. This is to ensure that neither the client nor the firm of solicitors end up out of pocket in the event of an unfavourable 'taxation'. Experts are usually able to obtain the fees they specify for their services, but even they will sometimes receive less than they had bargained for.

Apart from the very specialized area of forensic medicine referred to below, a number of doctors in a broad range of specialties are able to obtain regular amounts of expert medico-legal work. There is no obvious mechanism by which to enter this field. It is merely a question of experience gained over time, coupled with a willingness to make oneself available at very short notice (with all the inconvenience of frequently cancelled or adjourned hearings) and the active cultivation of relationships with firms of solicitors either locally, or if one has aspirations of higher things, with some of the specialist London firms.

The principal areas of civil litigation in which experts are required are:

- compensation for accident-related injury

- compensation for industrial disease

- compensation for medical negligence

- familial proceedings, eg involving child custody

- other financial litigation, eg where the state of mind of a patient is at issue.

The main problem with becoming a regular medico-legal expert lies in finding sufficient time to be available when solicitors or the courts require your services. For the busy consultant or GP it is not always a practical option. Writing reports is clearly within the expertise of most doctors, though the specialist medico-legal report is somewhat different and requires the exercise of medical judgement in a particular way. Giving evidence in court is, however, something which few doctors enjoy or excel at. Many doctors approach court appearances with horror and trepidation and consider the remuneration insufficient for the stress and inconvenience it involves.

Unfortunately the escalating cost of the judicial system has caused the government to seek to find ways of minimizing the costs involved. In the criminal sector, expert witness attendance fees can no longer be claimed from the solicitors but only from the court who will assess them in relation to the guidance rates published by the Lord Chancellor's Department (LCD) or the Crown Prosecution Service (CPS).

In civil cases, the availability of Legal Aid has become more limited but the amounts allowed for reports and witnesses are subject to even tighter controls so that the LCD's guidance rates are becoming a ceiling which few courts or taxing masters are willing to exceed. Nevertheless the amount of litigation and criminal proceedings shows no sign of abating and for the select few who take to such work it can be a stimulating and lucrative sideline.

The BMA publishes details of the LCD and CPS guidance rates. It also provides suggestions for fees for medico-legal work which is not publicly funded. However, it is expected that the majority of doctors in such situations will be obliged to negotiate their own fees, and that these fees will vary enormously depending on the circumstances of the case and the work required.

Forensic medicine

The recognition of forensic medicine as a fully fledged specialty is long overdue in this country, and it will not be long before it is officially recognized throughout the European Community. Opportunities to enter this field unfortunately are limited. There are three main areas of work: forensic pathology, which is mainly taken up with examination in the interests of justice of specimens from live or deceased victims or suspected perpetrators of crime;

forensic psychiatry, which involves examination of suspected or convicted criminals and their victims for judicial and/or therapeutic purposes; and forensic medical examination (or police surgeon) work.

Forensic pathologists may be NHS consultant pathologists on whole- or part-time contracts, or academics with university appointments. However, the bulk of forensic pathology (in England and Wales at least) is undertaken by Home Office-appointed forensic pathologists. These are highly trained and experienced individuals who have personally negotiated contracts with individual police forces to provide forensic pathology services making use of NHS or university facilities. Such individuals are not precluded from occasionally undertaking work for the defence in criminal cases. Standards of the work undertaken by Home Office appointees now come under the strict control of the Policy Advisory Board on Forensic Pathology.

Forensic psychiatrists are usually NHS or clinical academic consultants or occasionally psychiatrists of consultant status employed as senior prison medical officers. The remuneration of the former is likely to be an entirely ad hoc arrangement though it may be based on the rates laid down by the Committee for the Fees of Doctors Assisting Local Authorities (*see* below).

Police surgeons, or forensic medical examiners (FMEs) as they are known in certain parts of the country, occupy a curious position. Their responsibilities are principally medico-legal, ie in advising the police about the welfare of those in custody and undertaking physical examinations and taking samples of blood and urine from suspected criminals or alleged victims of crime in order to determine if a crime has been committed. On the other hand they have a duty of care to the occupants of police cells, victims of crime and to injured police officers, sometimes combining this with occupational health work for the police.

In discussions about the future of the police surgeon service, such as those which have been taking place recently in the Metropolitan Police area, all parties concerned have generally shied away from the notion of a full-time salaried service because this would tend to diminish, in the eyes of the public, the idea of the police surgeon being independent of the police. This independence is reinforced by the preservation of a system of payment based on item-of-service fees.

The level of individual fees and the mechanisms for payment are subject to a national agreement between the BMA, on behalf of the profession, and the Local Government Management Board, on behalf of the local authorities who are the paymasters of local police forces. The forum for discussion regarding these fees is a body calling itself the Joint Committee for the Fees of Doctors Assisting Local Authorities. Details of the payments agreed via this body can be obtained from either the BMA or the Local Government Management Board.

The changing nature of the judicial system is almost certain to bring about changes in the police surgeon service in the UK in the light of criticisms evidenced in the report of the Royal Commission on Criminal Justice. It is possible that such work will become subject to improved mechanisms of audit, with minimum standards of training, and that new mechanisms of payment may be devised in urban areas which will be more suitable to that kind of environment. Under the present system those working in urban areas with high levels of crime can, if they are prepared to devote a great deal of time to this often arduous and unpleasant work, earn considerable sums.

Almost all police surgeons are either active or retired GPs though there are a few consultants and other non-GPs among their number. In London many police surgeons are believed to be able to achieve amounts equal to GPs' average net remuneration with a few reported to be capable of earning over twice that amount. In rural areas the opportunities for police surgeon work are fewer and in some cases the additional income it provides may not amount to more than a few hundred pounds per annum.

Opportunities to become a police surgeon occur periodically. There is usually no other mechanism than to apply formally in writing to the local Chief Constable upon hearing of a vacancy. Fortunately there are frequent opportunities for GPs to familiarize themselves with the work by acting as locums for the regular police surgeons when they are unavailable. By this means it is usually possible to put oneself in a position whereby succession to a vacancy can be a formality. The situation will vary depending on location. In some areas there is a shortage of police surgeons and in others a surfeit. The Association of Police Surgeons (*see* Appendix) can provide more details of the work for those who are interested.

Occupational health

Occupational health is of course a recognized specialty and a great many of its practitioners will be full-time salaried employees of large companies or institutions. There may be several hundred such individuals. However there are probably a far greater number of part-time occupational physicians as the majority of firms will not find it necessary, practical or economical to employ a company doctor full-time. Small firms will prefer to employ a doctor, usually with some degree or knowledge of occupational health matters, on a sessional basis. In addition there are a small number of independent consultants in occupational medicine who may be called in by a firm to advise as an expert in some particular occupational health problem or problems. They may be paid on a short-term contract or item-of-service fee basis, subject to negotiation.

The BMA's Occupational Health Committee publishes suggested salary ranges for full- and part-time occupational physicians including suggested annual salaries based on one hour, two hours or one session (3½ hours) per week.

The duties which form the basis of the work vary considerably but broadly fall under two headings:

The effects of health on capacity to work

This involves:

- giving advice to employees on matters relevant to working capacity including medical examinations regarding initial placement, redeployment or retirement on health grounds

- providing immediate treatment for medical and surgical emergencies at the place of work

- examining and undertaking continued observation of persons returning to work after absence due to illness or accident, and giving advice about suitable work

- supervising the health of all employees

- giving advice to managers on provision of routine health surveillance and screening.

The effects of work on health

This involves:

- taking responsibility for first-aid services in accordance with the Health and Safety At Work Act, etc

- performing periodic examinations and medical supervision of persons exposed to special hazards in their employment

- giving advice to management about working environment and health risks, safety hazards and statutory requirements relating to health

- ensuring medical supervision of health and hygiene of staff facilities especially kitchens, canteens and production of food and drugs for sale to the public

- promoting educational work in respect of health, fitness and hygiene of employees.

The occupational physician occupies an unusual position vis-à-vis the employees of the company for whom he works and there is sometimes a danger, for instance, that the normal ethical rules of confidentiality will be in conflict with his responsibility to the company which employs him. Guidance on managing these conflicting responsibilities is available to BMA members in the following publications: *The Occupational Physician* and *Medical Ethics Today: Its Philosophy and Practice*.

Health screening

Health screening is now a familiar part of medical practice. While much of it occurs at places of work as part of company occupational health services and on the NHS, as part of GPs' health promotional activities, the market for private screening services had been buoyant until the economic recession of the early 1990s. The commercial sector continues to be dominated by BUPA which is the largest provider of screening services in Britain and Western Europe with (as of 1992) a network of 29 screening centres and 12 mobile units. Other major providers of screening services include BMI Healthcare (formerly AMI) which (as of 1992) had 12 screening centres; Private Patients Plan, with six screening centres in addition to a mobile screening operation (since taken over by BMI Healthcare); and Nuffield Hospitals. There were estimated to be 178 screening clinics in 1992. These varied widely from busy units to those open only for one or two sessions a week.

Much of the work of these screening centres is taken up with opportunistic screening of individuals. However a major part of their work is taken up with provision of check-ups of workers provided as part of special employee screening programmes developed for individual companies, or as part of joint union/industry initiatives, eg the electrical contracting industry's Joint Industry Board. There appears to have been recently a move away from the pioneering free-standing facilities towards private hospital-based screening clinics, frequently as part of joint ventures between hospitals and major providers of screening services. There is a considerable interest among women for self-pay screening for breast and cervical cancer, taking advantage of the limitations of the NHS screening services. Some health authorities are nevertheless developing screening services, eg private executive screening, as a means of income generation.

As regards work in the commercial sector, a few doctors are employed virtually full-time on a mixture of clinical and managerial duties. However, the vast majority work part-time on sessional contracts which usually comprise a retainer plus an amount for each patient seen. The work is interesting though usually undemanding. It seldom pays very highly and those who undertake such work usually do so because it is a regular commitment which can provide a mainstay when other ad hoc forms of private work dry up. Occupational physicians are foremost among those who undertake such work.

Insurance medicals

Insurance medical reports and examinations have for many years been a stable and not inconsiderable source of income for GPs. The amounts paid for life and permanent health insurance (PHI) reports and medicals are currently based on fees agreed by the BMA and the Association of British Insurers

(ABI). There are other forms of (general) insurance which sometimes require medical reports and examinations but with these other types, including travel insurance and, more often than not, health insurance, the patient/subscriber is required to meet the cost himself. Only with life assurance and PHI do the insurance companies agree to pay the negotiated rates (including 50% of the fee for a failed appointment). There is no agreed fee at present, however, for an HIV test (always a controversial subject of discussion in this context).

The staple of the insurance market is the personal medical attendant's (PMA) report, usually compiled from the GP's records. A higher fee is payable where a full physical examination is required, though this is almost always completed by an independent GP. It is possible for non-GPs to act as independent examiners for insurance companies, but the fees are modest and usually of little interest to consultants, and junior doctors do not usually have access to their own examination facilities.

In recent years, however, the GPs' monopoly of this particular market has come under fire from two sources: first from companies employing nurses and paramedics, and second from companies employing doctors, to undertake medicals in both cases at less than the BMA/ABI negotiated rates. Insurance companies have been tempted to make use of the services of such organizations, despite obvious concerns as to the quality of the service offered, because of the significant global costs of obtaining the medical evidence required for their business purposes. It is known that the insurance industry spends several million pounds a year on medical reports and examinations. It is doubtful, however, whether an alternative can be found for the PMA report which is an enormously valuable and unparalleled source of information about an individual's state of health and family medical history. Insurers in other developed countries would be envious of such a resource, which the medical examination can only supplement but never effectively replace.

Many GP practices currently make several thousand pounds a year from insurance-related work without much difficulty. Individuals with small patient lists, just starting out or concentrating on non-NHS work and who wish to obtain such work, can usually do so by writing to the major insurance companies detailing their experience, qualifications and availability. Insurance companies generally keep lists of doctors who have worked satisfactorily for them in the past whom they feel able to call on to undertake independent medical examinations in future.

Being aware of the threat posed to the GPs' monopoly of this work by companies employing nurses etc, certain enterprising organizations have set themselves up as intended intermediaries between GP practices and the insurance industry. It remains to be seen, however, whether these intermediaries are really able to guarantee the amount of work their advertising literature promises, as the major insurance companies generally continue to rely on their own approved lists of examiners.

Other forms of fee-paid work

Other forms of fee-paid work which are detailed in the BMA fees supplements include work for government departments, most notably examining medical practitioner or 'boarding' work for the Department of Social Security (Benefits Agency); sessional work for the Ministry of Defence or for the Department of Transport (Driver Vehicle Licensing Authority); part-time prison medical officer work for the Home Office Prison Service Department; sessional work for the Criminal Injuries Compensation Board; and work for the Health and Safety Executive's Employment Medical Advisory Service (EMAS) as an EMAS approved doctor undertaking medical examinations in relation to health and safety at work.

The fee supplements also detail various forms of sessional work in the Community Health Service and for local authorities under the Collaborative Arrangements (which deal with matters related to those authorities' statutory responsibilities in the fields of education, social services and public health); work as Visiting Medical Officers, to establishments maintained by local authorities or private nursing homes; school medical officer appointments; appointments as medical officers to football clubs, or 'crowd doctors' who officiate at a variety of sporting events; Medical Referees at Crematoria and various ad hoc services for local authorities governed by the Joint Committee for the Fees of Doctors Assisting Local Authorities, together with a host of 'miscellaneous' private services for which fees are usually payable by the patient. Advice and details of fees payable for all these areas of work are available to BMA members on request.

References and further reading

British Medical Association (1992) *Fees for Part-Time Medical Services*. (Guidance note).

British Medical Association (1991) *Medical Careers: A General Guide*. BMA, London.

British United Provident Association (1992) *A Guide to Private Consultant Practice*. BUPA, London.

Knight B (1993) *Legal Aspects of Medical Practice, 5th edn*. Churchill Livingstone, Edinburgh.

Medical Ethics Committee, BMA (1993) *Medical Ethics Today: Its Philosophy and Practice*. BMA, London.

Occupational Health Committee, BMA (1990) *The Occupational Physician*. BMA, London.

18

Conclusion: The Future of Private Medical Practice

The changing nature of private healthcare

At the beginning of this book it was claimed that the public and private healthcare systems were in many ways interdependent. The descriptions of GP and consultant practice, and of the operation of private hospitals and private medical insurance in subsequent chapters, have demonstrated this beyond the need for further explanation.

It therefore follows that any change in the prevailing medical culture or in the fundamental structure of the NHS will have a significant knock-on effect on its private-sector counterpart. We have noted that the reform of the NHS initiated by the Conservative government in the early 1990s represents the most radical shake up in the NHS since its inception. The changes wrought by these reforms have therefore had, and are continuing to have, a profound effect on the private sector.

One area in which these effects are discernible is in the relationship between GP and specialist. At the beginning of this book we noted that the GP/consultant relationship was crucial in both the NHS and the private sector. Referral to named specialists by the patient's GP is the common linchpin of both forms of healthcare provision. The introduction of fundholding has profoundly altered the relationship between GP and specialist in the NHS and its effects are being felt, in different ways, in the private sector. In the NHS it is clear that there has been an inexorable shift of power and influence from consultant to GP since the reforms were initiated. Regardless of how readily non-fundholding GPs take up the advice of the BMA in becoming involved in local purchasing decisions, it is clear that GPs as a class of practitioner carry considerably more clout than in bygone days. Accordingly, consultants as well as hospital business managers now recognize the need to consult with GPs on a regular basis about the provision of services. The increasing evidence of the custom whereby consultants work directly for GP fundholders in undertaking outpatient clinics at the GP's surgery (deemed by the Department of Health to be private practice for such consultants) is indicative of this changing relationship.

As regards the private sector, the GP fundholder is a potentially significant but presently unknown quantity. He remains, to use Laing's description, a 'wild card' in the calculation of private healthcare development. It is clear that many private hospitals were initially encouraged by the prospect of an upturn in business activity generated by GP fundholders seeking cheaper and speedier provision of elective surgery for their patients. However the natural conservatism of GPs has largely put paid to such expectations. There is no evidence yet of significant use of the private sector by fundholders. GPs do not seem to have diverged greatly from traditional referral patterns and are generally reluctant to take business away from their local provider units. Nevertheless the private sector continues to woo the powerful GP fundholder lobby, reassured by the encouraging noises from the government, which has recently removed all obstacles to the purchase by the NHS of private sector services where they prove cheaper or speedier.

Many commentators remain sanguine, however, about the prospects of fundholders transferring business to the private sector. Indeed there is actually a fear, expressed publicly by some health insurers, that some fundholders might seek to realise savings on their budgets by encouraging those of their patients who have private medical insurance to make use of their policies when elective surgery is required, something which fundholders themselves have vehemently denied.

GPs and health insurance

While GPs are being actively encouraged by the government to shop around for the best services and treatment for their NHS patients, there is as yet no evidence of them doing this for patients going private. The reason for this is simple: it is because the GP is unremunerated for his efforts in effecting referral to the private sector. He therefore has no incentive to shop around for 'best buys' for his patients seeking private-sector treatment.

The health insurers, as we have seen, have been trying, with mixed success, to introduce means of influencing the choice of specialist by their subscribers. Their efforts have been inhibited to some extent by their inability to make the GP a party to this process. The GP plays a vital role as initiator, facilitator and ultimately as judge of the outcome of private treatment yet, because he is unremunerated, he remains independent and cannot therefore serve as the instrument of the health insurers in containing the costs of specialist treatment. We have noted that this independence is, in other respects, of positive benefit to the patient and one must therefore weigh up the potential loss to the patient, against the benefit to the insurers, if GPs were permitted to be paid by a third party for their part in the proceedings.

One proposal put forward by Laing in his report on specialist fees for Norwich Union Healthcare was that GPs should be encouraged to refer to approved provider hospitals rather than to named specialists. This proposal faces two major obstacles: the fact that it runs counter to accepted practice within the NHS, and the fact that GPs have no incentive to diverge from the time-honoured practice of referral. The health insurers recognize that the GP's NHS terms of service continue to rule out appropriate financial provision for them in this process, yet the insurers have been strangely reluctant to increase the trifling amounts paid to GPs for validation of treatment, which many GPs erroneously regard as compensation for their time and trouble. Removing the bar to charging for private referral would necessitate a fundamental revision of the GP's terms of service, a move for which the Department of Health has so far shown no enthusiasm. It remains to be seen whether those advisers to the government who are anxious to encourage the development of the private sector will seek to tackle this as a means of removing a further obstacle to the level playing-field between the private and public sectors.

The use of audit and consumer expectations

We have already noted that the private sector is seeking to follow the lead of the NHS in making use of data derived from audit of specialists' activities. The health insurers are anxious to make use of the information available to NHS purchasers about waiting times, the range of services offered by provider units and the operating costs of many procedures in the NHS. What these purchasers do not have access to at present is information about how individual specialists perform and what the success rate of particular operations is between competing hospitals. This information does exist. Until recently it was confidential to the health departments and it was used only to identify those specialists whose standards of work fell below those of the best in their specialty, in order to bring about remedial retraining, and to identify hospitals whose services are below par in order to encourage by admonition and example, greater efforts at efficiency and adherence to 'best practice'.

In general the medical profession and the majority of health service administrators consider it inappropriate to publish such information. The medical profession is concerned at the quality of some of the audit data. They argue that its dissemination would moreover cause patients awaiting treatment unnecessary anxiety and demoralize those specialists whose performance was judged below average, and perhaps unjustly prejudice their professional standing; it would unjustifiably deter patients from being treated at local hospitals in some cases; and finally it might lay those hospitals and the specialists they employ open to an increased likelihood of medical negligence claims.

Many in the profession fear that the effect of this kind of competition would be to destabilize the present system and diminish the geographical spread of facilities, as patients are encouraged to travel greater distances in preference to, and to the detriment of, their local hospitals. In a fiercely competitive market, hospitals which cannot raise their standards (including NHS Trusts) may be forced to close, and it is a matter of debate whether this will be, in the best interests of the local population in the long term.

It has been noted that in certain parts of the USA such data are freely available and open to public scrutiny, resulting in the establishment of league tables of specialists and hospitals. Although this has been condemned by representatives of the medical profession both in the USA and the UK it is a sign of the pervasive influence of consumerism and of the Conservative government's commitment to market forces that, in late 1993, regional health authorities took the fateful step of allowing publication of waiting times for individual specialists and hospitals. It may not be very long before details of supposed success rates will be published also. The establishment of such specialist league tables will of course have a devastating effect for many specialists who, for often good reasons, may be unable to achieve the optimum success rates prescribed.

Some organizations presently advising the government would certainly welcome such developments and their views may be shared by many in the PMI industry. The insurers may feel their subscribers have a right to know whether the specialist to whom their GP proposes to refer them has a higher or lower than average success rate. But they will also wish to know for economic reasons. A higher risk of complications means potentially greater expense, and the future success of private medical insurance is considered by many in the industry to be dependent on lowering expenditure while increasing 'efficiency'.

The cost of specialist services and demand for PMI

Earlier we demonstrated that private healthcare in the UK is dominated by demand for private medical insurance. In any debate about the future of private healthcare, it follows that the price of PMI is all important. The early 1990s witnessed the growth of fierce competition among private medical insurers, as commercial companies entered the market until then dominated by the provident associations. To some extent this financial competition corresponded with a clash of competing ideologies. On the one hand there is the ideology of the established providents, sitting comfortably with a substantial, though diminishing, share of the corporate market, seemingly committed to support a system which aims to keep private medicine in the hands of a specialist elite able to guarantee high standards at high cost. On the opposite side of the fence there are the commercial insurers, new to this rarefied market place, restive at what they see as the restrictive practices of consultants, anxious to open up this previously finite market by making policies available to individual members of the public at low cost. To use a metaphor popular with economists, the commercials are unable to get a much bigger slice of the existing PMI 'cake' and so are anxious to make the cake bigger by creating new, cheap individual policies and so greatly expand the numbers of the public able to take advantage of them.

A major obstacle to the commercial insurers' attempts to bring down pricing is the cost of medical services. But why should the cost of medical fees be so important? After all, medical fees constitute only one third of the total costs of PMI expenditure, a proportion which has hardly changed in over 20 years. We have argued that it may be because medical fees are something of a soft target. That is not to say that the insurers have not tried to tackle hospital costs. We have noted the efforts made by all the major health insurers to bring down such costs by use of managed care initiatives. As one insurer put it, however, managed care is like squeezing a balloon—just as displacing air in one side of a balloon will cause it to expand on the other side, so measures like reducing the length of an in-patient stay will result in expenses being transferred to other areas, such as increased charges for drugs. Hospital costs are protean, whereas specialist fees present a stationary and identifiable target.

The MMC and the cost of specialist services

At the time this book went to press the final report of the Monopolies and Mergers Commission Inquiry had not yet been published. However, the MMC had already indicated that some 50% of NHS consultants were part of and benefited from what the Fair Trading Act 1973 defines as a 'complex monopoly situation'. The main reason for this finding was that some 9500 or so NHS consultants fixed more than 50% of their fees for private medical services in 1992 at or very close to the figures in either the BMA Guidelines or the BUPA or PPP schedules of procedures. Adherence to tariffs being adjudged to be anticompetitive, the Commission was then obliged to consider whether such practices were in the public interest.

Should the Commission consider that this monopoly is contrary to the public interest, there are a number of remedies which it can suggest to the Secretary of State for Trade and Industry. Included among these is the suppression of the BMA Guidelines.

It is clear that many in the health insurance industry might initially welcome this, believing that the Guidelines were inflationary in tendency and an obstacle to a free market. However, if, as suspected, the results of the MMC's survey show a greater convergence of specialists' fees around the BUPA maxima than the BMA Guidelines, then suppression of the latter would not in itself lead to a more open market and certainly not one as transparent as the public might wish.

At an early stage of the Inquiry the BMA expressed a willingness to become involved in the publication of information about specialist services which was directly and more accurately reflective of the full range of what specialists charge for individual procedures. The difficulty was in finding a means of obtaining the data necessary for such a publication and ensuring that its authenticity was not open to question. It will be interesting to see whether this suggestion features in the report of the MMC to the Secretary of State.

The Calman report and the supply of specialist labour

To add to their concerns at being unable to control the cost of specialist fees, a number of health insurers recognized that expansion of the market in private medical insurance could not be realized without a significant expansion in the numbers of specialists available to provide private treatment. Research by Laing and others has shown that NHS consultants cannot significantly increase the amount of private practice they are able to provide without detriment to their NHS responsibilities. They have shown consultants already undertake a significant amount of private practice during unsocial hours. Since all but a very small percentage of private practice is undertaken by specialists working partly or wholly for the NHS, only a significant increase in the number of NHS consultants could increase the supply of labour to facilitate an expansion of activity and, by increased competition among specialists, introduce internal pressures to reduce the cost of specialist services.

The number of consultants in the NHS is, however, strictly controlled in accordance with terms agreed between the government and the medical profession in the Department of Health's document *Hospital Medical Staffing: Achieving a Balance*, an agreement whereby the profession sought to balance the number of new consultant posts against the number of senior registrars likely to obtain specialist accreditation.

To some extent the health insurers have hamstrung themselves, in adhering closely to the terms of specialist accreditation laid down by the profession, and by recognizing the holding of an NHS consultant post as the touchstone of specialist recognition. There was effectively no way out of this particular dilemma, given the inevitable dependence on NHS specialists as providers of services to the private sector, until the publication of the Calman report into specialist accreditation.

No one should be mistaken about the implications of the recommendations of this working party for the future of both the NHS and private medicine. By recommending the reduction of the period of time necessary for completion of specialist training from an average of 10 to seven years, and making the award of the CCST as the official hallmark of specialist status, the Calman report threatens to create, at a stroke, an enormously expanded pool of specialist labour, as thousands of senior registrars eligible for the CCST suddenly become accredited and eligible for consultant posts within the NHS.

What the representatives of the profession are now grappling with in discussions with the health departments, is how the requisite number of new consultant posts can be created so as to provide jobs for these newly accredited specialists without abandoning altogether the delicate mechanism given expression in *Achieving a Balance*.

Effect of expanded manpower in the private sector

Of course the creation of this expanded pool of specialists may appear to offer what some of the health insurers have always wanted, but dealing with this new situation may pose further difficult questions for them. To begin with, will a new system whereby private treatment is delivered by less senior grades of doctor appeal to the public, accustomed to regard the personal service of the senior specialist as the distinguishing feature of private treatment? Many consultants currently undertaking private practice believe that it will result in a lowering of standards. But what effect would this have on demand for PMI? Just how readily will the health insurers, particularly those who benefit most from the present system, embrace the new system?

We have noted how closely the insurers have followed academic and clinical standards presented by the NHS. If the system which confines the right to undertake private practice to those trained to the present exacting standards is abandoned, will the health insurers likewise abandon their commitment to quality, or will they be tempted to find additional criteria in order to continue to exclude those whom they have not previously accredited? What has yet to be established in any event is the extent, if any, to which the health insurers, as private companies, are bound by EC directives. Some might argue that there is, in theory at least, no reason why the health insurers could not choose to implement a two-tier system of accreditation in order to weed out those whose training falls short of the optimum standards, whatever system the government chooses to institute for the NHS.

To many insurers and health economists the creation of more consultant posts and a new breed of specialist following Calman presents an opportunity. In his report *Private Specialist Fees: Is the Price Right?* William Laing speculated as to how the cost of medical fees could be curtailed. He listed various options, but the one he appeared to favour most was the direct employment by private hospitals of doctors having less experience than the present consultant grade, ideally on sessional contracts, or perhaps as full-time salaried employees. These doctors could be expected to work for salaries considerably below what their more senior colleagues can currently expect. If the government's previous record as regards creation of new consultant posts in accordance with the 2% per annum expansion stipulated in *Achieving a Balance* is anything to go by, the required number of new consultant posts may not materialize. In that case the army of newly qualified and unemployed specialists, their numbers swelled through restructuring of hospital services in

London in the wake of the Tomlinson report, will be immediately susceptible to the approaches of the private sector.

The appointment of full-time salaried specialists undertaking private surgical treatment exclusively in private hospitals would be the most radical departure from current norms of medical practice in the UK since the creation of the NHS. It may nevertheless provide the best means of achieving the level playing-field between the NHS and the private sector previously mentioned.

In this dual assault on the private specialist monopoly, that is to say the MMC Inquiry into private fees and the Calman review of specialist accreditation, the government has served as the instrument of change and the champion of those seeking to reform the private sector. The timing of this assault was presumably coincidental, though some would disagree. Some commentators have espoused a conspiracy theory whereby this is merely part of a wider hidden agenda through which the government hopes to dismantle the NHS and promote universal health insurance. This plan involves diminishing the public's reliance on the state health system by opening up the NHS to private sector competition and allowing the private sector to compete with the NHS on equal terms. As with all conspiracy theories the truth is probably far more mundane, yet there are many would-be government advisers advocating no less than what these conspiracy theorists maintain.

The NHS and the private sector: competitors or partners?

It is therefore ironic, perhaps, that at a time when the efforts of the government are working to the benefit of those seeking to reform the private healthcare sector, those efforts are, to a large extent, being undermined by the efforts to reform the NHS. For many years successive governments despaired of being able to put a ceiling on the escalating costs of the NHS and of being able to introduce reforms which would make it more efficient. The NHS has recently been transformed by the introduction of market forces and, most importantly, the purchaser/provider split. Whether the objectives for improvement set by the Conservative government in the early 1990s can ever be fully achieved remains to be seen. However, many in the private sector can be forgiven for hoping that they are not.

We have seen how important is the perception of waiting-lists to the uptake of private treatment. If waiting-lists are significantly reduced, as they are being in some areas, the uptake of private medical insurance may be reduced proportionally. 1992 saw a reduction in the number of subscribers to private medical insurance for the first time in many years. Although this was ascribed principally to the economic recession, it may also owe something to a subtle change in the perception of NHS provision on the part of the public at large.

Of even greater significance perhaps is the effect which the freedom to create new conditions of employment, which Trust hospitals now enjoy, is having on the availability of specialist manpower. Trust hospitals are already exercising their ability to prevent or restrict the ability of consultants employed on Trust contracts to undertake private practice outside Trust facilities. As Trusts organize their activities in a more businesslike manner it is inevitable that they will seek to maximize income by selling services direct to the private sector. In some cases they may do so by compelling their consultants to operate on private patients as part of their contractual duties, with the Trust taking all the private revenue derived therefrom from patients and health insurers.

While this will be unwelcome news for specialists it could be equally unwelcome for private hospitals who may thereby find the supply of labour, in the short term, drying up, while an increasing volume of private practice gravitates toward Trust hospital facilities with the connivance or approval of private medical insurers. The provision of 'hotel' service to NHS patients is already being actively encouraged in NHS hospitals as a means of generating extra income. To a large extent the provision of such services obviates some of the selling points of private treatment. At the same time NHS Trust hospitals are going all out to develop private facilities as a means of generating income necessary to subsidize other forms of treatment.

We have noted that Calman may eventually be viewed as the answer to the problem of specialist manpower availability in the private sector by ensuring that there is a greatly expanded pool of specialists. Yet it should not be assumed that the private sector will be the only beneficiary. Trust hospitals are just as anxious to make use of this new labour. If insufficient numbers of consultant posts are available to these newly qualified specialists, it is possible they will be happy to accept posts as Associate specialists, or perhaps as some new kind of 'intermediate' consultant not yet established, on the basis of personalized Trust contracts. The terms and conditions of such contracts would be greatly inferior to those enjoyed by consultants and would give the Trusts an unprecedented degree of control over their senior medical employees.

Nevertheless the range of work undertaken in NHS hospitals will be more demanding and therefore more appealing perhaps to the more dedicated specialist than the purely elective treatments carried out in private hospitals. The latter may therefore have to compete with Trusts if they are to try and obtain the services of full-time salaried specialists of the appropriate calibre and, once again, it is possible that Trusts may prove more than a match, in competitive terms, for the best that private hospitals can offer.

It may be argued that in this, as in other respects the aims of the NHS and the private sector are beginning to converge.

Recently the government itself implicitly recognized this by removing obstacles to private investment in NHS hospital facilities. There is a long history of partnership between the NHS and the private sector in certain specialized fields, eg pathology. The development of joint ventures in other fields may soon become commonplace. This may be viewed, from one point of view, as a move towards greater integration of the NHS and the private sector. There can be no doubt that this is the government's intention. It may turn out to be a very unequal partnership, however, for while the private sector waits for its moment of glory, the NHS is becoming leaner, more competitive and more businesslike as a result of the government reforms. It remains to be seen whether the private sector hospitals or NHS Trusts will be the greatest beneficiaries of the reform of the system of specialist accreditation.

The real impact of all the changes will not become apparent for many years to come. In the short term, many newly qualified specialists will be at liberty to undertake private practice in much the same way that their predecessors did. However, the changing expectation of patients in this consumerist society, coupled with the effects of the government-initiated reforms of the health service and abandonment of alleged restrictive practices in the private sector, will undoubtedly ring the changes to an unprecedented extent, perhaps before those specialists reach the peak of their medical careers.

Until recently, it was possible to plan one's career as a specialist in terms of increasing or diminishing amounts of private practice, particularly as one approached and passed retirement from the NHS. Unfortunately, as this brief foray into possible future developments suggests, specialists may no longer be able to predict with any certainty what the future may hold for them in private practice.

References and further reading

Blair P and National Economic Research Associates (1993) *Healthcare Report: Reforming the Private Sector*. Norwich Union Healthcare, Norwich.

Calman K (1993) *Hospital Doctors: Training for the Future—Report of the Working Group on Specialist Medical Training*. DoH, London.

Laing W (1992) Healthcare Report: *UK Private Specialists' Fees—Is the Price Right?* Norwich Union Healthcare, Norwich.

Laing W (1993) *Laing's Review of Private Healthcare 1993*. Laing & Buisson, London.

UK Health Departments/Joint Consultants Committee/Chairmen of Regional Health Authorities (1988) *Hospital Medical Staffing: Achieving a Balance*. DoH, London.

Appendix

Useful Addresses

Provident associations

Bristol Contributory Welfare Association (BCWA)
Bristol House
40–56 Victoria Street
Bristol BS1 6AB
Tel: (0272) 293742

British United Provident Association (BUPA)
Provident House
Essex Street
London WC2R 3AX
Tel: (071) 353 5212

Civil Service Medical Aid Association
Princess House
Horace Road
Kingston upon Thames
Surrey KT1 2SL
Tel: (081) 547 1555/974 5432

Exeter Hospital Aid Society
Beech Hill House
Walnut Gardens
Exeter
Devon EX4 4DG
Tel: (0392) 75361/2

Private Patients Plan (PPP)
PPP House
Crescent Road
Tunbridge Wells
Kent TN1 PL
Tel: (0892) 512345

Private Patients (Anglia) Ltd
124 Thorpe Road
Norwich
Norfolk NR1 1RS
Tel: (0603) 629504

Provincial Hospital Services Association (PHS)
44 Harpur Street
Bedford
Bedfordshire MK40 2QU
Tel: (0234) 267371

Western Provident Association (WPA)
Rivergate House
Blackbrook Park
Taunton
Somerset TA1 2PE
Tel: (0823) 623000

Commercial insurers

Ambassador Insurance Company Ltd
205 Brooklands Road
Weybridge
Surrey KT13 0PE
Tel: (0932) 821056

Avon Insurance
Arden Street
Stratford upon Avon CV37 6WA
Tel: (0789) 415415

Cigna Employee Benefits
PO Box 42
Greenock
Renfrewshire PA15 4AZ
Tel: (0475) 892224

Eagle Star Insurance Company Ltd
The Grange
Bishops Cleeve
Near Cheltenham
Gloucestershire GL52 4XX
Tel: (0242) 221311

Iron Trades Insurance Company Ltd
Huntingdon House
10 Mason's Hill
Bromley
Kent BR29 JWA
Tel: (081) 313 1000

London & Edinburgh Insurance Group
The Warren
Worthing
West Sussex BN14 9QD
Tel: (0903) 820820

MGI Prime Health
Wey House
Farnham Road
Guildford
Surrey GU1 4XS
Tel: (0483) 440 550

NFU Mutual
Tiddington Road
Stratford upon Avon
Warwickshire CV37 7BJ
Tel: (0789) 204211

Norwich Union Healthcare Ltd
Chilworth House
Hampshire Corp Park
Templars Way
Eastleigh
Hampshire SO5 3RY
Tel: (0703) 266533

OHRA UK Ltd
17 East Links
Tollgate Industrial Estate

Chandlers Ford
Hampshire SO5 5YR
Tel: (0703) 620620

Orion Insurance Company Plc
Orion House
Bouverie Road West
Folkestone
Kent CT20 2RW
Tel: (0303) 850303

Pinnacle Insurance Company Ltd
Premier House
Elstree Way
Borsham Wood
Hertfordshire WD6 1DH
Tel: (081) 953 4433

PPP Medicalcare Ltd
111 Chertsey Road
Woking
Surrey GU21 5BW
Tel: (0483) 740000

Provincial Insurance Plc
Stramongate
Kendal
Cumbria LA9 4BE
Tel: (0539) 723415

Strasbourgeoise Assurance Mutuelle
90 Sloane Street
London SW1X 9PQ
Tel: (071) 259 5260

Sun Alliance Insurance Group
Richmond House
Richmond Hill
Bournemouth
Dorset BH2 6EQ
Tel: (0202) 292464

Third party administrators

Allied Medical Assurance
18 Buckingham Gate
London SW1E 6LB
Tel: (071) 630 0533

Executive Healthcare
Radio House
John Wilson Business Park
Whitstable
Kent CT5 3QP
Tel: (0227) 772666

Healthcare Management Ltd
Winterton House
Nixey Close
Slough
Berkshire SL1 1NG
Tel: (0753) 512500

Healthcare Agencies Ltd
18 Buckingham Gate
London SW1E 6LB
Tel: (071) 630 0533

Hogg Robinson Gardner Mountain
Imperium
Imperial Way
Reading
Berkshire RG2 0UD
Tel: (0734) 758000

Managed Care Consultants Ltd
Crossways House
39 East Street
Epsom
Surrey KT17 1BL
Tel: (0372) 748090

Medisure Marketing & Management Ltd
17 Portland Square
Bristol
Avon BS2 8FJ
Tel: (0272) 429331

Remedi Health Management Services
Hogg Robinson House
42–62 Greyfriars Road
Reading
Berkshire RG1 1NN
Tel: (0734) 583683

Willis Healthcare
1 St John's Gate
Valpy Street
Reading
Berkshire
Tel: (0734) 596067

Hospital operators: commercial

Bourn–Hallam
112 Harley Street
London W1N 1AF
Tel: (O71) 631 1583

BUPA Hospitals Ltd
15 Essex Street
London WC2R 3AX
Tel: (071) 379 1111

Charter Medical of England
11/19 Lisson Grove
London NW1 6SH
Tel: (071) 258 3828

Community Hospitals Group Plc
Priory Terrace
24 Bromham Road
Bedford
Bedfordshire MK40 2QD
Tel: (0234) 273473

Compass Healthcare Ltd
Queen's Wharf
Queen Caroline Street
London W6 9RJ
Tel: (081) 741 4441

Country Care Homes Ltd
Whitecliffe Nursing Home
14 East Park Road
Blackburn
Lancashire BB1 8AT
Tel: (0254) 681491

Cygnet Healthcare Plc
Godden Green Clinic
Godden Green
Sevenoaks
Kent TN15 0JR
Tel: (0732) 63491

Galen Health Care Inc
Wellington Place
London NW8 9LE
Tel: (071) 586 5959

General Healthcare Group Plc
4 Cornwall Terrace
Regents Park
London NW1 4QP
Tel: (071) 486 1266

Goldsborough Ltd
Techno House
Low Lane
Horsforth
Leeds
West Yorkshire LS18 4DF
Tel: (0532) 591177

Great Northern Health Management Ltd
4 Cornwall Terrace
Regents Park
London NW1 4QP
Tel: (071) 486 1266

Hospital Corporation International Group Plc
25 Windsor Street
Chertsey
Surrey KT16 8AY
Tel: (0932) 569166

Independent British Hospitals Ltd
3rd Floor
Prudential House
Topping Street
Blackpool
Lancashire FY1 3AX
Tel: (0253) 23901

Independent Care Management
26 Eccleston Square
London SW1V 1NS
Tel: (071) 630 8001

International Care Services Ltd
Ashlyns Hall
Berkhamsted
Hertfordshire HP4 2ST
Tel: (0442) 863301

International Hospitals Group Ltd
Stoke Park
Stoke Poges
Slough
Berkshire SL2 4NS
Tel: (0753) 73222

Nestor Medical Services Ltd
15 Southampton Place
London WC1A 2BU
Tel: (071) 404 3122

Paracelsus-Kliniken
Parkside Hospital
53 Parkside
Wimbledon
London SW19 5NX
Tel: (081) 946 4202

Priory Hospitals Group
Priory Lane
Roehampton
London SW15 5JJ
Tel: (081) 878 9559

The Rehabilitation Group Ltd
Huntercombe Lane South
Taplow
Maidenhead
Berkshire SL6 0PQ
Tel: (06286) 67881

Sister Rose Ltd
Knowle House
Sagars Road
Handforth
Cheshire SK9 3ED
Tel: (0625) 530792

St Martins Hospitals Ltd
97–99 Park Street
London W1Y 3HA
Tel: (071) 409 3112

United Medical Enterprises Ltd
Old Bank House
High Street
High Wycombe
Buckinghamshire HP11 2AN
Tel: (0494) 473773

Hospital operators: charitable

British Pregnancy Advisory Service
Austy Manor
Wooton Wawen
Solihull
West Midlands B95 6BX
Tel: (05642) 3225

Nuffield Hospitals
Nuffield House
1–4 The Crescent
Surbiton
Surrey KT6 4BN
Tel: (081) 390 1200

Population Services FPP Ltd
108 Whitfield Street
London W1P 6BE
Tel: (071) 388 0662

Screening clinic operators

BMI Healthcare Health Services Division
4 Cornwall Terrace
Regents Park
London NW1 4QP
Tel: (071) 486 1266

BUPA Medical Centre Ltd
Battle Bridge House
300 Grays Inn Road
London WC1X 8DU
Tel: (071) 837 6484

Nuffield Hospitals
Nuffield House
1–4 The Crescent
Surbiton
Surrey KT6 4BN
Tel: (081)390 1200

PPP Medical Centre Ltd
99 New Cavendish Street
London W1M 7FQ
Tel: (071) 637 8941

Wellcare (UK) Health Screening Franchises Ltd
7 Monmouth Place
Bath
Avon BA1 2AU
Tel: (0225) 447048

Pathology laboratory operators

BUPA Hospitals Ltd
15 Essex Street
London WC2R 3AX
Tel: (071) 379 1111

Cambridge Management & Marketing Ltd
Kingfisher House
7 High Green
Great Shelford
Cambridge
Cambridgeshire CB2 5EG
Tel: (0223) 845841

Cleveland Medical Laboratories Ltd
Letch Lane Carlton
Stockton on Tees
Cleveland TS21 1EE
Tel: (0642) 673737

General Healthcare Group Plc
4 Cornwall Terrace
Regents Park
London NW1 4QP
Tel: (081) 486 1266

JS Pathology Plc
Bewlay House
32 Jamestown Road
London NW1 7BY
Tel: (071) 267 2672

Occupational health service providers

BMI Healthcare Health Services Division
2nd Floor
Cottrell House
53/63 Wembley Hill Road
Wembley
Middx HA9 8DL
Tel: (081) 903 2222

BUPA Occupational Health
Unit 3
Parsonage Business Park
Parsonage Way
Horsham
West Sussex RH12 4AL
Tel: (0403) 65020

General Medical Clinics
67 Wimpole Street
London W1N 7DE
Tel: (071) 636 5145

Minerva Health Management Ltd
283 High Street
Berkhamsted
Hertfordshire HP4 1AJ
Tel: (0442) 870011

PPP Corporate Health Services
99 New Cavendish Street
London W1M 7FQ
Tel: (071) 637 8941

Financial advisers and brokers

BMA Services Ltd
Freepost
Tavistock House South
Tavistock Square
London WC1H 9BR
Tel: (071) 387 4311

General Practice Finance Corporation
Tavistock House North
Tavistock Square
London WC1H 9JL
Tel: (071) 387 5274

Medical Insurance Agency
166 Plymouth Grove
Longsight
Manchester
M13 0AH
Tel: (061) 273 5354

Relevant organizations

Association of Anaesthetists of Great Britain and Ireland
9 Bedford Square
London WC1B 3RA
Tel: (071) 631 1650

Association of British Insurers
51 Gresham Street
London EC2V 7HQ
Tel: (071) 600 3333

Association of Police Surgeons of Great Britain
Creaton House
Creaton
Northamptonshire NN8 8ND
Tel: (060) 124722

British Association of Dermatologists
7 John Street
London WC1N 2ES
Tel: (071) 404 0092

British Association of Otolaryngologists
Royal College of Surgeons
35–43 Lincoln's Inn Fields
London WC2A 3PN
Tel: (071) 242 7750

British Association for Rheumatology and Rehabilitation
41 Eagle Street
London WC1R 4AR
Tel: (071) 405 8573

British Healthcare Association
24a Main Street
Garforth
Leeds LS25 1AA
Tel: (0532) 320903

British Medical Association
BMA House
Tavistock Square
London WC1H 9JP
Tel: (071) 387 4499

Department of Health/Department of Social Security
Richmond House
79 Whitehall
London SW1 2NS
Tel: (071) 210 3000

Faculty of Anaesthetists
Royal College of Surgeons
35-43 Lincoln's Inn Fields
London WC2A 3PN
Tel: (071) 405 3474

Faculty of Dental Surgery
Royal College of Surgeons
35–43 Lincoln's Inn Fields
London WC2A 3PN
Tel: (071) 405 3474

Faculty of Occupational Medicine
Royal College of Physicians
11 St Andrew's Place
London NW1 4LE
Tel: (071) 935 1174

Faculty of Ophthalmologists
35–43 Lincoln's Inn Fields
London WC2A 3PN
Tel: (071) 405 6754

General Medical Council
44 Hallam Street
London W1N 6AE
Tel: (071) 580 7642

Independent Doctors Forum
67 Wimpole Street
London W1M 7DE

Independent Healthcare Association
22 Little Russell Street
London WC1A 2HT
Tel: (071) 430 0537

Joint Committee on Higher Medical Training
Royal College of Physicians
11 St Andrews Place
London NW1 4LE
Tel: (071) 935 1174

Joint Committee on Higher Psychiatric Training
Royal College of Psychiatrists
17 Belgrave Square
London SW1X 8PG
Tel: (071) 235 2351

Joint Committee on Higher Surgical Training
Royal College of Surgeons
35–43 Lincoln's Inn Fields
London WC2A 3PN
Tel: (071) 405 3474

Medical Defence Union
3 Devonshire Place
London W1N 2EA
Tel: (071) 486 6181

Medical and Dental Defence Union of Scotland
Mackintosh House
120 Blythswood Street
Glasgow G2 4EH
Tel: (041) 221 5858

Medical Practices Committee
1st Floor
Eileen House
80–94 Newington Causeway
London SE1 6EF
Tel: (071) 972 2930

Medical Protection Society
50 Hallam Street
London W1N 6DE
Tel: (071) 637 0541

Monopolies and Mergers Commission
New Court
48 Carey Street
London WC2A 2JT
Tel: (071) 324 1467

National Association of Health Authorities and Trusts
Birmingham Research Park
Vincent Drive
Birmingham B15 2SQ
Tel: (021) 471 4444

Royal College of General Practitioners
14 Princes Gate
Hyde Park
London SW7 1PU
Tel: (071) 581 3232

Royal College of Obstetricians and Gynaecologists
27 Sussex Place
Regents Park
London NW1 4RG
Tel: (071) 262 5425

Royal College of Pathologists
2 Carlton House Terrace
London SW1Y 5AF
Tel: (071) 930 5861

Royal College of Physicians
11 St Andrews Place
London NW1 4LE
Tel: (071) 935 1174

Royal College of Physicians and Surgeons of Glasgow
242 St Vincent Street
Glasgow G2 5RJ
Tel: (041) 221 6072

Royal College of Physicians of Edinburgh
9 Queen Street
Edinburgh EH2 1JQ
Tel: (031) 225 7324

Royal College of Psychiatrists
17 Belgrave Square
London SW1X 8PG
Tel: (071) 235 2351

Royal College of Radiologists
38 Portland Place
London W1N 3DG
Tel: (071) 636 4432

Royal College of Surgeons of Edinburgh
Nicolson Street
Edinburgh EH8 9DW
Tel: (031) 556 6206

Royal College of Surgeons of England
35–43 Lincoln's Inn Fields
London WC2A 3PN
Tel: (071) 405 3474

Scottish Council for Postgraduate Medical & Dental Education
12 Queen Street
Edinburgh EH2 1JE
Tel: (031) 225 4365

Scottish Home and Health Department
Establishment Division
St Andrews House
Regent Road
Edinburgh EH1 3DG
Tel: (031) 556 8400

Society of Occupational Medicine
11 St Andrews Place
London NW1 4LE
Tel: (071) 486 2641

Start as You Mean to Go On: The Consultant's Practical and Financial Guide to Private Practice is obtainable by writing to:
G.K. Elliot
42 Cheryls Close
Bagley Lane
London SW6 2AY

Index